养生保健法：
逆转疾病及老化

李永正 医学士　　李永仁 医学士

李应绍 医学博士/心脏学博士
　　　　副教授、心脏内科及老人医学专科指导医师

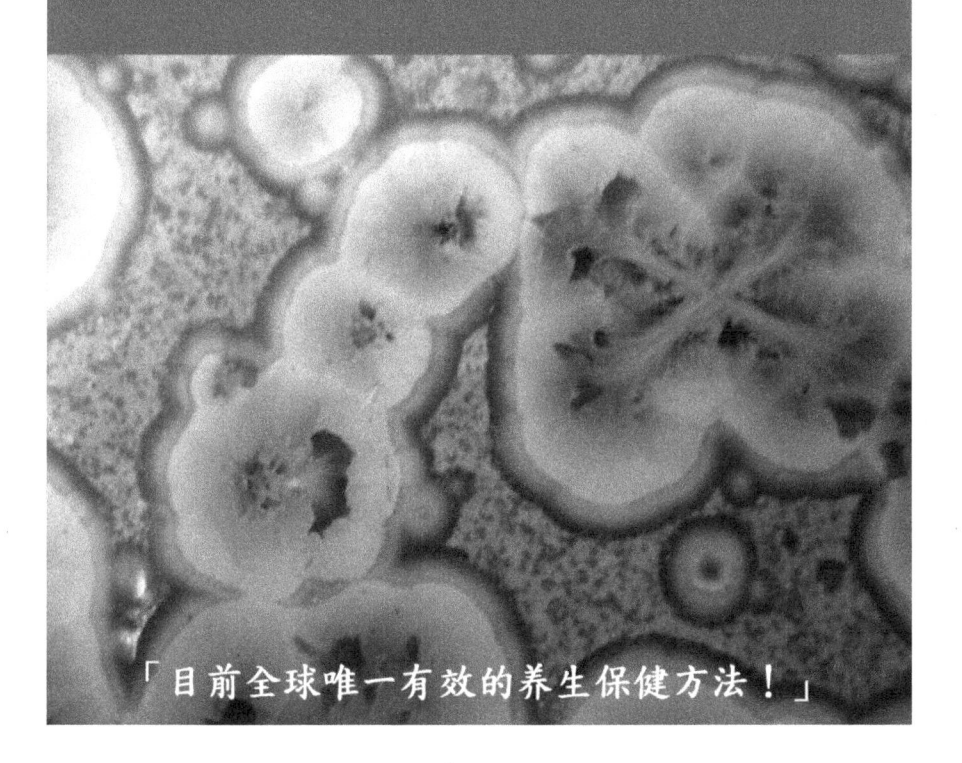

「目前全球唯一有效的养生保健方法！」

划时代!

医界証实的养生保健法!

真正让您健康!

本书不是坊间文章! 是医学论文!

是目前全球唯一有效的养生保健方法!

Copyright © 2023 David Wing-Ching Lee, William Wing-Ho Lee and Andrew Ying-Siu Lee
All rights reserved.
ISBN: 9786267105344
No part of this book may be reproduced or transmitted in any form or by any means, including photocopy, recording, or any information storage and retrieval system, without permission in writing from the authors.
IngramSpark Publishing
Printed in the United States of America

医学知识在不断变化。尽管作者认为本书中所述的药物选择和剂量以及设备和装置的规格和使用符合出版时的当前建议和惯例，但作者对本书所描述的信息不做任何保证。在这本书中，鉴于正在进行的研究，设备开发，政府法规的变化以及与生物医学有关的数据的快速积累，强烈建议读者仔细阅读和评估本书提供的信息。

本书提供医界证实的养生保健法，眞正让您健康！

自100多年前以来，老少连体动物实验证明，可以逆转疾病和老化。血液或血浆交换输血以及年轻（或正常）因子的供给和年老（或异常）因子的同时去除，也会产生这种现象。

最近报导，与老少连体实验相似，心脏优化会产生心脏保护性（或正常）因子。配合健康的飲食，规律运动，健康的生活方式，全身系统优化（自愈机能）是一种自然的养生保健法，可以逆转疾病和老化。

还包括有关传统及近期养生保健法，衰老和抗衰老的主题。本书适合一般民众，病患和医护专业人员。人人都渴望健康！

前言

医生忙于治疗疾病，而花较少的时间来做卫教或让患者咨询有关养生保健法的知识。此外，临床医生倾向于将重点放在药物和器械疗法上，而往往忽视利用养生保健法来预防，治疗甚而逆转疾病和衰老。本书的主要目的是提供有关养生保健法的充分信息，以便全世界的人都可以将其纳入正在进行的医疗保健中，通过逆转疾病，而获得更長的健康期，和通过逆转老化，而达到命定的生命期。医护专业人员可能还会发现这本书有助于教育患者。俗话说，目标不是增加寿命，而是增加生命品质。

本书是我今年发表的医学论文完整版，其标题为："Heart conditioning and heterochronic parabiotic models as healthy strategies"（SN Comprehensive Clinical Medicine 5:6,2023）。本书有中英文(Healthy regimen: reversion of disease and aging, Amazon Publishing,2021. https://www.amazon.com/dp/B09LGGSSGR?ref_=pe_3052080_397514860) 两种版本。我希望有很多人能仔细通读这本书，遵守适当的养生保健法，获得更長的健康期和生命期，并享受健康美好的生活。健康是指您没有疾病，也没有老化。养生保健，就是逆转疾病及老化。

知识就是力量。人人有权获得知识。本书旨在迎合不同级别的所有读者。它介绍了有关养生保健法的一般及专业知识,适合民众,病患(了解一般知识及专业概念)和医护专业人员(学习或复习专业知识)。

养生保健～ 关乎生命生活～ 必须学习～ 必须实行～

李应绍 医学博士/心脏学博士
副教授、心脏内科及老人医学专科指导医师
台中仁爱综合医院
www.heartdisease.idv.tw

目 录

第一章 传统养生保健法
1.1 健康饮食 13
1.2 规律运动 26
1.3 健康生活方式 36
1.4 健康指引 42
1.5 预防医学 46

第二章 近期养生保健法
2.1 压力（stress）、双相剂量效应（hormesis）、平衡等稳性（homeostasis） 53
2.2 心脏优化 57
2.3 肺优化 70
2.4 肠优化 78
2.5 全身优化 92
2.6 再生医学 96
2.7 纳米医学 105
2.8 氧气疗法 111
2.9 益生菌、益菌生、益生菌合并剂 123
2.10 植物营养素 129
2.11 荷尔蒙替代疗法 136
2.12 抗氧化剂 141
2.13 另类医学 147

第三章 老化及抗老化

3.1 老化 161

3.2 抗老化 176

第四章 养生保健法：逆转疾病及老化　　189

第一章

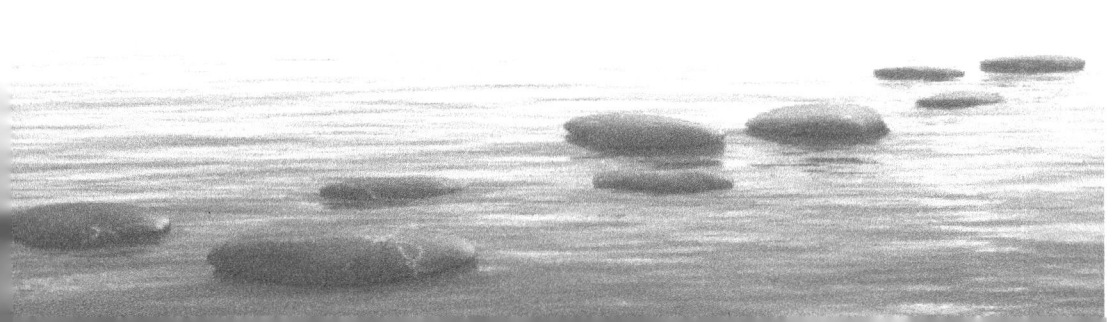

传统养生保健法

1.1 健康饮食

饮食在整体健康和生命品质中起着重要作用。为了身体的健康和正常功能，人类需要食用作为能量和营养物质的食物和饮料。此外，饮食可以预防和治疗诸如肥胖，高血压，糖尿病，心血管疾病，癌症，过敏，骨质疏松，胃肠道和免疫疾病等疾病。

如今，随着城市化和经济增长，饮食结构的变化导致卡路里消耗的增加和整体饮食质量的下降。快餐食品是不健康的饮食，具有高卡路里含量，大量加工肉，高度精制的碳水化合物，含糖饮料和不健康脂肪。超市还取代了当地的新鲜食品和农家店，并成为高度加工食品，高热量小吃和含糖饮料的来源。

现在，健康饮食被定义为最大限度地延长健康和延长寿命的饮食。健康饮食由碳水化合物，蛋白质和脂肪，水以及多种维生素，矿物质和微量元素组成。这些多量营养素 (macronutrient) 和微量营养素 (micronutrient) 不仅能提供能量，而且还能促进细胞的生长，维持和修复。过多或过量食用可导致健康状况不佳或与营养有关的发病率和死亡率。

多量营养素被大量食用并提供大量能量。三种主要的多量营养素包括碳水化合物，蛋白质和脂肪。

碳水化合物应占总卡路里摄入量的 45-65%。碳水化合物的质量可以通过对碳水化合物的血糖反应（血糖水平）来评估，例如血糖指数 (glycemic index) 和血糖负荷（glycemic load，血糖指数与食物中碳水化合物含量的乘积）。低血糖指数食品包括蔬菜，坚果，豆类和谷物。高血糖指数食品包括土豆，糖果，白面包和其他由谷物制成的精制产品。高血糖指数的饮食具有罹患糖尿病，冠状动脉疾病和癌症的高风险[1,2,3]。

蛋白质应占总卡路里摄入量的 10-35%。富含蛋白质的健康食品包括鱼类，家禽，瘦肉，鸡蛋，豆类，豌豆，豆制品，坚果和种子。红肉和加工肉类食用量的增加与糖尿病，中风，结肠直肠癌和心血管疾病的风险增加有关[4]。食用动物产品时，选择鱼，家禽，奶制品和鸡蛋。通常选择植物蛋白作为主要来源[5]。

脂肪应占总卡路里摄入量的 20-35%。饱和脂肪 (saturated fat) 和反式脂肪 (trans fat)（例如肉，

奶酪，人造奶油，烘焙食品，快餐和冰淇淋）会导致心血管疾病，而单饱和脂肪 (monosaturated fat) 和多不饱和脂肪 (polyunsaturated fat)（例如鱼，橄榄油，坚果）则具有相对保护作用。应用含有单饱和和多不饱和脂肪的油烹饪，例如玉米，橄榄油和花生油。脂肪的质量比总脂肪的摄入量更为重要，并且相对于动物脂肪而言，偏爱植物性脂肪的饮食更为有益[6]。Omega-3 和-6 脂肪是多不饱和脂肪。鱼，坚果，低芥酸菜籽油，绿色蔬菜中的 Omega-3 脂肪以及橄榄油，坚果和鳄梨中的单不饱和脂肪具有健康益处。玉米和植物油是 omega-6 脂肪。

微量营养素的需求量非常小，其中包括多种矿物质和维生素。矿物质仅占典型人类饮食的 5%，但对正常健康和功能至关重要。矿物质被归类为需求量大矿物质，其中包括成年人每天需要摄入含量超过 100 毫克的矿物质，例如钠，钾，钙，镁和磷。微量元素是成年人每天所需含量为 1-100 毫克的矿物质，例如铜，氟化物，碘，锰，锌。超微量元素是成年人每天所需少于 1 毫克的矿物质，例如铬，硒和砷。钠的高摄入量与高血压和心血管疾病，中风，胃癌和肾脏疾病有关。钙和维生素 D 是正常骨骼等稳性和功能所必需的。抗氧化剂维生素包括维生素 A，C，E 和

β-胡萝卜素。许多食物，尤其是水果和蔬菜都含有这些维生素。

综合维生素补充剂可考虑用于存在维生素缺乏症风险的患者，例如酗酒者，水果和蔬菜摄入量低的低质量饮食，吸收不良，纯素食，血液透析患者等。除非有特定的适应症，否则不建议在健康饮食摄入足够量的人补充综合维生素和矿物质来预防慢性疾病，因为缺乏有效的临床证据。健康成年人中也没有必要进行维生素血液水平测试，只有在临床上怀疑维生素缺乏症时才应考虑进行测试，例如在确定的骨质疏松症评估中测量维生素 D 和钙水平。

水果和蔬菜富含纤维，必需的维生素和矿物质以及低血糖指数的碳水化合物。水果和蔬菜摄入量的增加与心血管疾病，中风，癌症及死亡率的风险降低相关 [7,8]。建议每餐的一半由蔬菜和水果组成。绿叶蔬菜具有最大的健康益处。

豆类包括各种豆类，这些豆类的纤维，蛋白质，铁，维生素和矿物质含量高，且血糖指数低 [9]。食用豆类食物可减少心脏和脑血管疾病，延长寿命，改善血糖控制和改善体重管理 [9,10]。

膳食纤维的摄入与降低心脏病，糖尿病和癌症的风险有关。纤维的良好来源包括全谷物，水果，蔬菜和豆类。

乳制品由牛奶和奶制品（例如奶酪，酸奶）组成。乳制品是蛋白质，钙，维生素 D 和钾的良好来源。乳制品可降低罹患心血管疾病，中风和癌症的风险[11]。

水是仅次于空气的第二大生命必需品。生物的主要成分是水。水可能是最重要和有益的饮料。水对于温度调节，酸碱平衡，运输，内源性和外源性物质的排泄至关重要，并促进许多生理机能，这对人体等稳性至关重要[12]。建议成年人每天喝 1.5 升的总水量，包括从饮料和食物中摄取的水，并针对活动较大个体和对液体敏感的医疗状况的患者进行调整[13,14]。

水的来源范围很大，包括自来水，过滤或开水，瓶装水，井水或其他。理想情况下，饮用水应仅包含水分子。水中发现的任何生物，物理，化学或放射性物质都称为污染物。细菌，病毒和寄生虫等微生物污染物会在数小时或数天内引起疾病。其他污染物，例如化学和矿物质，农药和化肥，重金属，会在多

年后引起疾病。如果您发现颜色，气味或味道有所变化，请检查饮用水的质量。许多人饮用瓶装水或过滤水是因为它具有纯净的优势。

不建议喝碳酸饮料和其他含糖饮料。这些饮料是饮食中精制糖和卡路里的主要来源，因此是体重增加和肥胖的关键因素。酒精会增加患乳腺癌，口腔癌，食道癌，喉癌，咽癌和肝癌；其他疾病，例如肝硬化和酒精中毒的风险。咖啡因是世界上消耗最多的兴奋剂，通常是指咖啡和茶。根据现有数据，没有足够的临床证据来推广或阻挠日常饮食中的咖啡和/或茶消费。

盐是一种常见的调味剂，会增加患高血压和心脏病的风险[15]。

世界卫生组织（World Health Organization，WHO）关于健康饮食的建议强调减少饱和和反式脂肪酸，糖和盐的摄入，同时增加水果，蔬菜，坚果和全谷类的摄入。

低脂饮食，低碳水化合物饮食，素食饮食，DASH饮食和地中海饮食是维持良好健康的最常用饮

食方式。所有这些饮食方式都与健康有益。

地中海饮食 (Mediterranean diet) 通常富含水果，蔬菜，全谷类，豆类，坚果和种子，其中橄榄油是重要的脂肪来源。它通常包括少到中量的鱼，家禽和奶制品，几乎没有红肉。

DASH （Dietary Approaches to Stop Hypertension，控制高血压的饮食）的饮食富含水果和蔬菜，纤维含量高，低脂日常饮食，脂肪含量适中，动物蛋白含量低，饱和脂肪含量低，并且含有许多植物蛋白，包括豆类和坚果。

低碳水化合物生酮饮食 (ketogenic diet) 已用于减轻体重，癫痫，糖尿病，心血管疾病和神经系统疾病数十年。经典的生酮饮食是一种高脂肪、充足蛋白质、低碳水化合物的饮食，会导致血液中酮、胰岛素、葡萄糖、胰高血糖素和游离脂肪酸的代谢变化。生酮饮食应由营养师监督，一般建议实行至少三个月，最长两年。

在过去的几十年中，世界各地的人们体重和肥胖增加了，这主要是饮食结构变化和运动水平下降的

结果。高血压，糖尿病，高脂血症，肥胖，癌症的风险随着体内过多脂肪的增加而增加，并且体重指数（body mass index，BMI）和腰围增加[16,17]。

BMI 可以简单地通过体重（公斤）除以身高 BMI 可以简单地通过体重（公斤）除以身高平方（米）来计算。正常体重是 BMI 18.5 – 24.9 Kg / m2。超重是 BMI 为 25-29.9 Kg / m2，肥胖是 BMI 大于 30 Kg / m2。体重不足的体重指数低于 18.5 公斤/平方米。除了测量 BMI 之外，还测量了超重和肥胖成年人的腰围，以评估腹部肥胖 (abdominal obesity)。男性腰围大于 40 英寸（102 厘米），女性腰围大于 35 英寸（88 厘米），表示心脏、新陈代谢风险增加[18]。腹部肥胖的患者罹患心血管疾病，糖尿病，高血压，血脂异常的风险更高，并且总体死亡率较高[19]。在临床评估中，应同时监测 BMI 和腰围。研究表示，与腰围相关的风险要比高 BMI 的风险更强[20]。调整饮食以维持正常的 BMI 和腰围非常重要。如果您超重，请少吃。如果体重不足，请多吃。食用的碳水化合物类型和数量可能对健康产生重要影响。强调低碳水化合物或无碳水化合物的饮食已成为减轻体重的流行方法。

高血压是全世界死亡的主要危险因素，甚至超过香烟，高血糖，高脂和肥胖。饮食对于有效预防，治疗和控制高血压起著至关重要的作用。富含水果，蔬菜，豆类和低脂乳制品的饮食，而少摄入零食，糖和肉类的饮食（例如地中海和 DASH 饮食）可降低血压并预防高血压和心血管疾病。

体重过重是糖尿病最重要的危险因素。富含全谷物食品，水果和蔬菜且总脂肪（尤其是动物脂肪）含量低的饮食可以预防糖尿病。

约 70% 的成年人有营养风险或营养不良[21]。营养不良与死亡风险增加相关[22]。常规补充综合维生素和矿物质并不建议，除非老年人饮食的总摄入量低，否则可能无益[23]。

慢性病是全球发病率和死亡率的主要原因[24,25]。饮食控制在许多疾病过程的病因和演变中发挥作用。长期以来，已知饮食控制可以预防，减缓甚至逆转某些疾病过程，尤其是肥胖症和糖尿病。据估计，健康饮食包括蔬菜，水果，全谷类，鱼类和减少红肉，动物脂肪和精制糖的摄入量，可预防 30-35%的癌症[26]。饮食控制也可以改善癌症治疗结果[27]。

地中海饮食可减少认知能力下降，老人痴呆症或阿兹海默氏病 (Alzheimer's disease)。

　　总体而言，健康饮食在促进健康和预防疾病方面起著核心作用。健康饮食习惯是一种健康的生活方式。健康饮食方式代表了摄入所有食品和饮料的总量。可以改善饮食质量和健康结果，并减少与饮食相关的疾病风险。

参考文献

1. Bhupathiraju SN, Tobias DK, Malik VS et al. Glycemic index, glycemic load, and risk of type 2 diabetes: results from 3 large US cohorts and an updated meta-analysis. Am J Clin Nutr 2014; published online April 30. DOI:10.3945/ajcn113.079533
2. Dumesnil JG, Turgeon J, Tremblay A et al. Effect of a low-glycemic index-low fat-high protein diet on the atherogenic metabolic risk profile of abdominally obese men. Br J Nutr 2001;86:557
3. Franz MJ, Bantle JP, Beebe CA et al. Evidence-based nutrition principles and recommendations for the treatment and prevention of diabetes and related complications. Diabetes Care 2002:25:148
4. Pan A, Sun Q, Bernstein AM et al. Red meat consumption and risk of type 2 diabetes: 3 cohort of US adults and an updated meta-analysis. Am J Clin Nutr 2011;94:1088-96
5. Song M, Fung TT, Hu FB et al. Association of animal and plant protein intake with all cause and cause-specific mortality. JAMA Intern Med 2016;176(10):1453-63
6. Hu FB, Van Dam RM, Liu S. Diet and risk of type II diabetes: the role of types of fat and carbohydrate. Diabetologia 2001;44:805-17
7. Miller V, Mente A, Dehghan M et.al. Fruit, vegetable, and legume intake, and cardiovascular disease and deaths in 18 countries(DURE): a prospective cohort study. Lancet 2017;390:2037
8. HeFJ, Nowson CA, MacGregor GA. Fruit and vegetable consumption and stroke: meta-analysis of cohort studies. Lancet 2006;367:320
9. Messina V. Nutritional and health benefits of dried beans. Am J Clin Nutr 2014;100(suppl 1):437S-442S
10. Papanikolaou Y, Fulgoni VLIII. Bean consumption is associated with greater nutrient intake, reduced systolic

blood pressure, lower body weight and a smaller waist circumference in adults: results from the National Health and Nutrition Examination Survey 1999-2002. J Am Coll Nutr 2008;27(5):569-76
11. Elwood PC, Pickering JE, Hughes J et al. Milk drinking, ischemic heart disease and ischemic stroke II. Evidence from cohort studies. Eur J Clin Nutr 2004;58:718
12. Riveros-Perez E, Riveros R. Water in the human body: An anesthesiologist's perspective on the connection between physicochemical properties of water and physiologic relevance. Ann Med Surg 2018;26:1-8
13. Valtin H. Drink at least eight glasses of water a day. Really? Is there scientific evidence for 8 x 8 ? Am J Physiol Regul Integr Comp Physiol 2002;283:993-1004
14. Juan WY, Basiotis P. More than one in three older Americans may not drink enough water. Nutrition Insights. United States Department of Agriculture 2002.
15. He FJ, Li J, Macgregor GA. Effect of longer-term modest salt reduction on blood pressure. Cochrane Database Syst Rev 2013;4:CD004937
16. Adams KF, Schatzkin A, Harris TB et al. Overweight, obesity and mortality in a large prospective cohort of persons 50 to 71 years old. N Eng J Med 2006;355:763
17. Renehan AG, Tyson M, Egger M et al. Body mass index and incidence of cancer: a systematic review and meta-analysis of prospective observational studies. Lancet 2008;371:569
18. Jensen MD, Ryan DH, Apovian CM et al. 2013 AHA/ACC/TOS guideline for the management of overweight and obesity in adults: a report of the American College of Cardiology/American Heart Association Task Force on Practice Guidelines and The Obesity Society. Cir 2014;129:S102
19. Guatinc L, Algre-Diaz J, Wade R et al. General and abdominal obesity and mortality in Mexico City: Prospective study of 150000 adults. Ann Intern Med 2019

20. Vazquez G, Dural S, Jacobs DR Jr, Silventoinen K. Comparison of body mass index, waist circumference, and waist/hip ratio in predicting incident diabetes: a meta-analysis. Epidemiol Rev 2007;29:115-28.
21. De Luis D, Lopex Guzman A, Nutritional Group of Society of Cstilla-Leon (Endocrinology, Diabetes and Nutrition). Nutritional status of adult patients admitted to internal medicine departments in public hospitals in Castilla y Leon, Spain-A multi-center study. Eur J Intern Med 2006;17:556
22. Wallace JI, Schwartz RS, LaCroix AZ et al. Involuntary weight loss in older outpatients: incidence and clinical significance. J Am Geriatr Soc 1995;43:329
23. Mursu J, Robien K, Harnack LJ et al. Dietary supplements and mortality rate in older women: the Iowa Women's Health Study. Arch Intern Med 2011;171:1625
24. Global Burden of Disease Study 2013 Collaborators. Global, regional and national incidence, prevalence and years lived with disability for 301 acute and chronic diseases and injuries in 188 countries, 1990-2013: a systemic analysis for the Global Burden of Disease Study 2013. Lancet 2015;386:743-800
25. GBD 2013 Mortality and Causes of death Collaborators. Global, regional and national age-sex specific all-cause and cause-specific mortality for 240 causes of death, 1990-2013: a systematic analysis for the Global Burden of Disease Study 2013. Lancet 2015;385:117-71
26. Wick A, Hagmann J. Diet and cancer. Swiss Med Wkly 2011;141:w13250
27. Saleh AD, Simone BA, Palazzo J et al. Calorie restriction augments radiation efficacy in breast cancer. Cell cycle 2013;12(12):1955-63

1.2 规律运动

强烈建议规律运动是预防慢性疾病和保持健康的最有效方法之一[1]。与吸烟，高血压和糖尿病等已确定的危险因子相比，少活动的生活方式可能是发病率和死亡率更强有力的预测指标[2]。缺乏运动与心血管疾病和中风，肥胖，糖尿病，癌症，骨质疏松症，阿兹海默氏病 (Alzheimer's disease) 和帕金森氏病 (Parkinson's disease) 等多种疾病的发病率增加有关。

身体活动是任何持续的骨骼肌肉身体运动，例如步行，慢跑，跳舞，游泳等，与休息相比，会增加能量消耗。运动是指定期进行有计划的，有目的的和重复性的体育活动，以改善或维持健康和体适能。运动可以分为四种主要类型：

一、有氧运动（aerobic exercise），例如：步行或跑步。是指「有氧需求」，是指肌肉从血液中需求足够的氧气以维持长时间活动的运动。它涉及大肌肉群的连续和有节奏的运动，会使心率增加，呼吸变得更加困难，这可以增加心血管和呼吸的适应性。

二、无氧运动（anaerobic exercise），是指「无氧需求」。又称为力量（strength）或抗力（resistance）运动。例如举重，向上拉，向上推，下蹲等。这种运动让肌肉从血液中获取的氧气不足以维持长时间的活动，它涉及短暂的重复性肌肉收缩，可以增加肌肉力量。

三、脚后跟步行或太极拳等平衡运动（balance exercise），可改善平衡感和本体感觉。

四、活动性或柔韧性运动（mobility or flexibility exercise），如伸展运动或瑜伽之类的运动，可以改善关节的活动能力。

在运动过程中应该同时进行所有四种运动类型是非常重要的。

运动计划应从 5 到 10 分钟的热身运动开始（缓慢的有氧运动，如缓慢行走，伸展运动和柔韧性运动）。热身运动可以使心率逐渐增加，并可以减少受伤的风险。然后混合有氧运动，力量运动，平衡运动和活动性或柔韧性运动，以保持运动计划的乐趣和趣味性。运动锻炼后，应进行 5 分钟的伸展运动或轻度有氧运动来休息。运动计划应该令人愉快，以鼓励长期运动的承诺。运动没有针对特定年龄的心率建

议，不需达到特定心率仍可获得健康益处。如果您感到呼吸困难，疲倦和出汗，那您就已经足够努力了。

建议每周五天至少进行 30 分钟的中等强度有氧运动（例如快步走）。或者，建议每周三天进行 20 分钟的强度有氧运动（例如慢跑）。避免连续两天不进行体育锻炼。如果您不能连续运动 30 分钟，请尝试一次运动 10 分钟左右，每天 3 到 4 次。即使运动时间较短，对您也有好处。没有适合所有人的运动计划。总的来说，鼓励绝大多数人开始温和的运动计划，并逐步发展到可以接受的更有活力的运动计划。

任何运动计划都应设计成适合参与者的健康和身体状况。还应考虑和评估参与者现有的医疗状况，年龄和喜欢的运动类型。

没有慢性病（例如心脏病，糖尿病，肾脏疾病）或涉及症状（如胸部不适，呼吸困难，头昏眼花）的人通常在进行运动计划之前不需要进行医学检查评估。患有严重疾病或症状的患者应在进行运动计划之前进行临床评估。此外，当患者病重时，应避免运动。

规律运动的好处远大于潜在的风险。肌肉骨骼损伤是最常见的运动风险。为了安全地进行运动并避免出现问题，请确保在运动期间和运动后多喝水，并选择安全，通风良好，不要太热，太冷或太湿的运动环境。最好在饭前一小时进行运动（对于糖尿病患者，饭后一小时），如果您年纪大，体弱或生病，则必须有同伴。如果您有胸痛或胸闷，恶心或呕吐，心慌，头晕或昏厥，请停止运动并咨询医生，尤其是症状持续或恶化超过 10 分钟时。

规律运动对健康有益。规律运动可降低各种原因和特定疾病的发病率和死亡率的风险[4]。规律运动在至少 26 种医学疾病的治疗中起着重要作用，包括心血管疾病，中风，高血压，糖尿病，癌症[5]。因此，经常运动是最好的药物之一，应该更广泛地使用。

超重和肥胖的人减轻体重可以降低心血管和糖尿病的风险。运动会导致临床上显著的体重减轻，从而导致葡萄糖体内等稳性，并改善心脏新陈代谢危险因子，例如体脂肪，内脏脂肪，脂质，胰岛素敏感性[6,7]。运动可降低血压[8]，降低心血管疾病和中风的风险[9]。运动可改善血管内皮功能和自主神经功能，对

缺血性心脏病和心律不整具有保护作用[10]。此外，运动在糖尿病的预防和治疗中也起着重要作用[11]。体育活动还可以预防或延迟其他长期糖尿病并发症的发生，例如神经系统，视网膜和肾脏的病理，并可能减慢现有疾病的进展及并发症[12]。

血小板，高水平的血浆纤维蛋白原（plasminogen activator inhibitor，PAI-1）活性，组织型纤溶酶原激活物（plasminogen activator，t-PA）抗原和血浆黏度升高在心血管和脑血管疾病的发病机理和进展中起着重要作用。运动可减少血小板粘附和聚集[13]，降低 PAI-1 活性和 t-PA 抗原[14]，降低血浆粘度[15]，并改善纤溶活性(fibrinolytic activity)[16]，因此改善与血栓形成相关的止血因子，并预防缺血性心脏病和脑中风。

运动可以调节脑细胞的形成，大脑新陈代谢和大脑血管的形成，因此有益于脑功能和健康[17]。运动可改善睡眠，压力和焦虑，抑郁[18]和认知功能[19]。

规律运动可增强疫苗接种反应，减少疲惫/衰老的免疫 T 细胞数量，增加 T 细胞增生能力，降低发炎

细胞因子 (inflammatory cytokines)，增加白血球吞噬(防御)活性，降低对感染的发炎反应，增强免疫 NK 细胞的防御活性和更长的白血球染色体端粒长度 (抗老化引起)，所有这些都表示，经常运动可以随着年龄的增长而调节和改善免疫系统并延缓免疫衰老的发生 (immunosenescence，免疫系统功能下降) [20]。

运动有益于各个年龄段的人，并可能降低全因发病率并延长寿命[21]。进行一些规律运动总比没有好，并且从事规律运动永远不会太晚。老年人运动的主要好处包括改善整体健康状况，改善体能，柔韧性，活动性和适应性，可以改善日常功能，帮助保持独立性并降低跌倒和跌倒相关伤害的风险[22]。规律运动可以延缓老化过程，并减轻与年龄有关的疾病的隐患。运动可维持有氧运动能力，肌肉质量和肌肉强度[23]。运动对骨密度，大小和形状具有有益的作用，改善骨质疏松症和骨骼健康[24]。运动可增强抗氧化防御机制[25]。运动有益于运动功能，步态，认知功能和神经退化性疾病，例如阿兹海默氏病和帕金森氏症[26,27]。缺乏运动会增加十种以上癌症的风险[28]。运动

可以预防乳腺癌，肠癌，肾癌，肺癌，胃癌等癌症[18,28]。此外，规律运动与癌症相关的主要预后有关，包括生活质量[28]。

参考文献

1. Latimer-Cheung AE, Toll BA，SP。Promoting increased physical activity and reduced inactivity. Lancet 2013;381(9861):114
2. Ross R, Blair SN, Arena et al. Importance of assessing cardiorespiratory fitness in clinical practice: a case for fitness as a clinical vital sign: a scientific statement from the American Heart Association. Cir 2016;134:e653.
3. Thompson PD, Franklin BA, Balady GJ et al. Exercise and acute cardiovascular events placing the risks into perspective; a scientific statement from the American Heart Association Council on Nutrition, Physical activity and Metabolism and the Council on Clinical Cardiology. Cir 2007;115:2358.
4. Kodama S, Saito K, Tanaka S et al. Cardiorespiratory fitness as a quantitative predictor of all-cause mortality and cardiovascular events in health men and women: a meta-analysis. JAMA 2009;301:2024
5. Pedersen BK, Saltin B. Exercise as medicine – evidence for prescribing exercise as therapy in 26 different chronic diseases. Scand J Med Sci Sports 2015;25(suppl3):1-72.
6. Donnelly JE, Honas JJ, Smith BK et al. Aerobic exercise alone results in clinically significant weight loss for men and women : Midwest exercise trial 2. Obesity 2013;21:E219-228.
7. Wallberg-Henriksson H, Zierath JR. Metabolism. Exercise remodels subcutaneous fat tissue and improves metabolism. Nat Rev Endocrinol 2015;11:198-200.
8. Brook RD, Appel LJ, Rubenfire M et al. Beyond medications and diet; alternative approaches to lowering blood pressure: a scientific statement from the American heart association. Hypertension 2013;61:1360
9. Owen N, Sparling PB, Healy GN et al. Sedentary behavior: emerging evidence for a new health risk. Mayo Clin Proc 2010;85:1138

10. Sixt S, Rastan A, Desch S et.al. Exercise training but not rosiglitazone improves endothelial function in pre-diabetic patients with coronary disease. Eur J Cardiov Prev R 2008;15:473-8.

11. Hayes C, Kriska A. Role of physical activity in diabetes management and prevention. J Am Diet Assoc 2008;108:S19-S23.

12. Boule N, Haddad E, Kenny G, Wells G, Sigal R. The effects of exercise on glycemic control and body mass in type 2 diabetes. JAMA 2001;286:1218-27.

13. Wang JS, Jen CJ, Chen HI. Effects of exercise training and deconditioning on platelet function in men. Arterioscler Thromb Biol 1995;15:1668

14. Stevenson ET, Davy KP, Seals DR. Hemostatic, metabolic and androgenic risk factors for coronary heart disease in physically active and less active postmenopausal women. Arterioscler Thromb Vas Biol 1995;15:669

15. Levine GN, O'Malley C, Belady GJ. Exercise training and blood viscosity in patients with ischemic heart disease. Am J Cardiol 1995;76:80

16. Killewich LA, Mack RF, Montgomery PS et al. Exercise training enhances endogenous fibrinolysis in peripheral arterial disease. J Vasc Surg 2004;40:741

17. Cotman CW, Berchtold NC, Christie LA. Exercise builds brain health : key roles of growth factor cascades and inflammation. Trends Neurosci 2007;30(9):464-72.

18. Piercy KL, Troiano RP, Ballard RM et al. The physical activity guidelines for Americans. JAMA 2018;320:2020

19. Loprinzi PD, Kane CJ. Exercise and cognitive function: a randomized controlled trial examining acute exercise and free-living physical activity and sedentary effects. Mayo Clin Proc 2015;90:450

20. Simpson RJ, Lowder TW, Spielmann G, Bigley B, LaVoy EC, Kunz H. Exercise and the aging immune system. Ageing Res Rev 2012;11:404-20.

21. Martinez-Gomez D, Guallar-Castillon P, Garcia-Esquinas E et al. Physical activity and mortality in older community-dwelling women. J Am Geriatr Soc

22. Miller ME, Rejeski WJ, Reboussin BA et al. Physical activity, functional limitations and disability in older adults. J Am Geriatr Soc 2000;48:1264

23. Booth FW, Lees SJ. Fundamental questions about genes, inactivity and chronic disease. Physiol Genom 2007;28:146-57.

24. Fontana L, Meyer TE, Klein S, Holloszy JO. Long-term low-calorie low-protein vegan diet and endurance exercise are associated with low cardiometabolic risk. Rejuvenation Res 2007;10:225-34.

25. Mota MP, Peixoto FM, Soares JF et al. Influence of aerobic fitness on age-related lymphocyte DNA damage in humans: relationship with mitochondria respiratory chain and hydrogen peroxide production. Age 2010;32:337-46.

26. Santes-Lozano A, Pareja-Galeano H, Sauchis-Gomar F et al. Physical activity and Alzheimer disease; a protective association. Mayo Clin Proc 2016;91:999-1020.

27. da Silva FC, Iop R da P, de Oliveira LC et al. Effects of physical exercise programs on cognitive function in Parkinson's disease patients: a systemic review of randomized controlled trials of the last 10 years. PLoS One 2018;e0193113.

28. Gaskin CJ, Craike M, Mohebbi M et.al. Association of objectively measured moderate-to-vigorous physical activity and sedentary behavior with quality of life and psychological well-being in prostate cancer survivors. Cancer Causes Control 2016;27:1093-103.

1.3 健康生活方式

健康生活方式通常与您可以服用的任何药物一样有效，甚至更有效。如果饮食正确，规律运动，避免吸烟和饮酒，则不太可能出现各种健康问题。

吸烟是导致过早患病和死亡的主要可避免原因。戒烟的好处仅在几个月后就开始显现，并在数年内达到不吸烟者的利益，即使对于老年人也是如此。因此，戒烟永远不会太晚。吸烟还增加了患糖尿病的风险，戒烟可以通过减少全身性炎症来降低糖尿病的风险。

选择健康的饮食方式，例如 DASH 或地中海饮食，而不是偏向于特定的喜爱食品，可以减少糖尿病的发生。

健康的生活方式，包括饮食调整，减轻体重和规律运动，可以减缓糖尿病的进展，并降低心血管疾病和总死亡率。生活方式的改变通常是有益的，不会产生不利影响。健康的生活习惯是必要的，例如，避免在工作或在家中承受压力，饮食健康，进行规律运

动和保持积极的心理态度，保持智力和身体活动，当然还要避免致癌物质，尤其是烟草。此外，社会互动对健康和长寿有很大影响。不幸的是，衰老常常伴随着社交互动的减少。这可能是由于我们自己的行为随着年龄的增长，失去亲戚朋友，退休等而发生的变化。

总体而言，建议对生活方式进行以下调整：

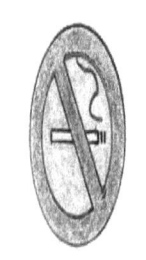

不抽烟 — 香菸有：尼古丁(-->心肌梗塞)，焦油(致癌)，一氧化碳(=毒气体-->缺氧)。每抽一根菸-->**减五分钟寿命**

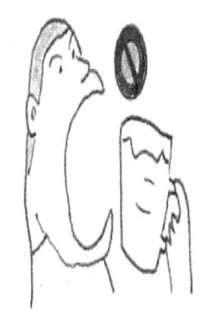

不喝酒 — 喝酒伤害肝、胰及心脏。并导致神经紧張，癌，脑血管病等

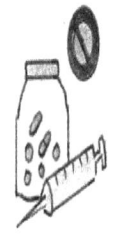

避免毒素 — 不吸毒，不滥用药品，避免环境毒素如铅、二手烟、废气、辐射、微波等

不过日夜颠倒
夜生活
早睡早起 — **自律神经失调**

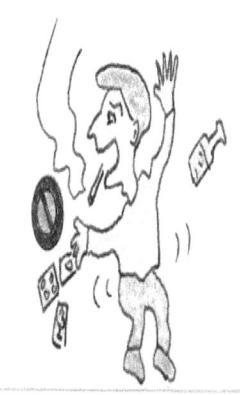

健康生活方式

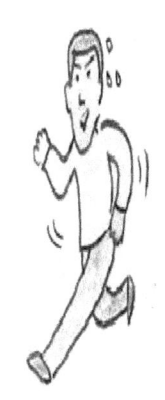

適当规律运动 — 可改善血压,血糖,血脂肪。增加骨质密度,心肺功能,体力,免疫力。预防老化,癌症等

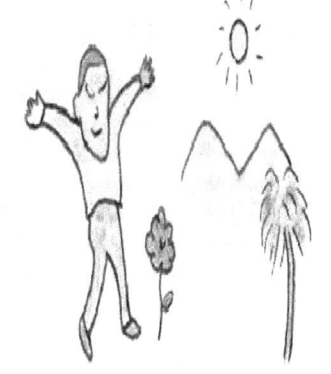

適当休闲 避免工作过劳 — 调節神经,内分泌,心血管,消化道功能。减少压力緊張。

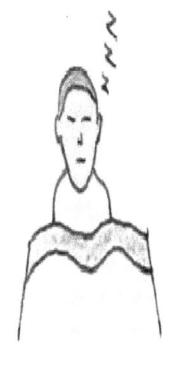

睡眠均衡
- 睡眠6-8小時。过度或不足都不好
- 午睡15-30分钟。太久会影响晚间睡眠
- 就寝前4小时的睡意要忍耐(若此時睡 --> 晚間睡不好)
- 睡眠促进脑功能,抗老化,免疫,充分休息

健康生活方式

每天早上顺畅排便习惯。不憋尿		促进排泄功能
適量吃肉，蛋，油脂，水果(均衡饮食，不偏食)		肉类含优质胺基酸，可提升免疫力，制造骨骼，肌肉。蛋含优质胺基酸，DHA，卵磷脂，矿物質，可强化骨骼，脑，肌肉及内脏组织。油脂是合成荷尔蒙及细胞膜成分，是身体必需营养素。
不暴饮暴食，吃八分饱，少量多餐，少吃零食，晚餐也少吃一些		可降低血糖，改善肥胖
多咀嚼		能促进消化、吸收。预防牙周病、蛀牙、動脈硬化、肥胖、失智症、老化及癌症

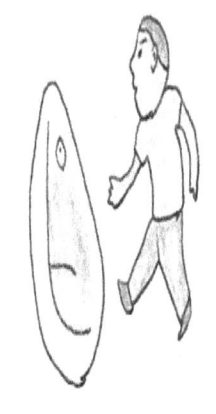

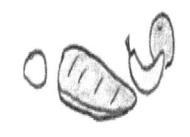

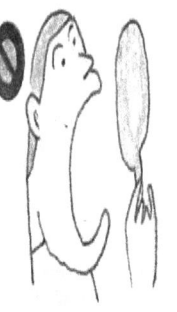

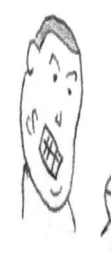

健康生活方式

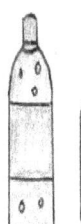

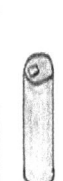

少喝饮料 — 饮料含糖及盐分-->高血压，动脉硬化，肥胖，糖尿病，免疫力下降

自信、乐观、情绪、欢笑、爱心、保持快乐心态 — 可改善压力、内分泌、自律神经、血糖、免疫力

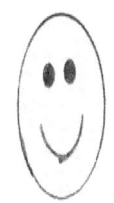

良好个人性格，处事能力，人际关系，社交活动，积极应对，适应社会环境。避免精神紧张，心烦意乱，忧郁寡欢，易受刺激，平衡心理 — 心理不健康（=重要致病因素）

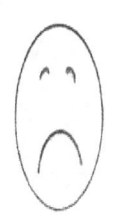

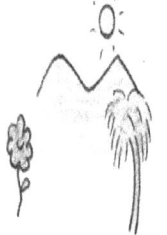

良好生活自然环境，卫生习惯 — 阳光，空气，水，噪音，绿化等生态及卫生环境

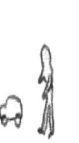

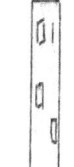

良好社会环境 — 经济、文化、风俗、教育、治安、居住、工作、家庭环境

健康生活方式

1.4 健康指引

健康饮食指引[1]：-

1. 遵循健康的饮食习惯，在适当的卡路里水平内摄入所有食品和饮料。 也就是说，富含蔬菜，水果，全谷类，海鲜，豆类，坚果的饮食，中等含量的低脂或脱脂乳制品，含量较低的红肉和加工肉，含量较低的甜味食品和饮料以及精制谷物，限制饱和脂肪，添加糖和盐。 健康的饮食习惯可以促进整体健康，并降低罹患心血管疾病，超重和肥胖，糖尿病，癌症，认知障碍，痴呆，阿兹海默病，抑郁症的风险；并预防骨质疏松症和骨折，并提高骨矿物质密度。

2. 注意食品多种类，营养品质和份量

3. 限制糖，饱和脂肪，反式脂肪和盐的摄入量

4. 转向更健康的食物和饮料选择

5. 达到并保持正常体重

6. 不饮酒的人不得以任何理由开始饮酒。

规律运动指引[2]：

1. 规律运动促进正常的生长和发育，使人感觉和功能更好，并减少许多慢性疾病的风险。数月和数年的规律运动可以产生长期的健康益处。

2. 成人规律运动关键准则：
   - 成人应整天活动而少坐。有运动总比没有好。
   - 成人每周应至少进行 150 分钟的中等强度的运动，或每周进行 75 分钟的剧烈强度的有氧运动
   - 成人还应该每周 2 天或更多天进行中等强度或更高强度的 肌肉增强活动

3. 老年人的规律运动关键准则：
   - 成人规律运动关键准则也适用于老年人。
   - 老年人应进行多部分运动，包括有氧运动，肌肉增强和平衡 运动。
   - 老年人应根据自己的健康水平来调整自己的运动强度。

- 患有慢性病或残疾的老年人应在医疗保健提供者的照料下，在其能力和状况允许的情况下安全地进行规律运动。

健康生活方式指引[3]：-

1. 预防心血管疾病的最重要方法是终生实行健康的生活方式。

2. 所有成年人都应饮食健康，并达到及保持正常体重。

3. 所有成年人应至少进行 150 分钟的中等强度的规律运动或每周 75 分钟的剧烈强度的规律运动。

4. 戒菸，避免接触二手烟。

参考文献

1. US Department of Health and Human Services; US Department of Agriculture. 2015-2020 Dietary Guidelines for Americans. 8th ed. Washington, DC: US Dept of Health and Human Services; December 2015. https://health.gov/dietaryguidelines/2015/guidelines
2. US Department of Health and Human Services. Physical Activity Guidelines for Americans. 2nd ed. Washington, DC: US Dept of Health and Human Services;2018.
3. Arnett DK, Blumenthal RS, Albert MA et al. 2019 ACC/AHA guideline on the primary prevention of cardiovascular disease: a report of the American College of Cardiology/American Heart Association Task Force. JACC 2019;74(10):e177-232

1.5 预防医学

大多数人宁愿永不生病，或者如果无法避免疾病，则他们希望在疾病造成任何伤害之前及早发现。即，早期发现和早期治疗。为了做到这一点，就算没有特别症状的健康人会接受定期检查，以识别和避免危险因素，从而避免疾病发生或在病程中及早发现疾病，以便早期治疗预防疾病。这便是预防保健，预防健康检查或预防医学。

临床预防医学有四种主要类型：接种疫苗 (immunization)，筛检 (screening)，改变生活方式 (lifestyle modification) 和药物预防 (chemoprevention)。所有这四种类型在一生中都适用。

接种疫苗可以预防儿童早期的某些疾病。成人接种疫苗包括白喉，百日咳和破伤风，以及预防流感，肺炎球菌性肺炎，甲型和乙型肝炎的预防接种[1]。

筛检是在疾病开始引起症状或问题之前对无症状未病，有害状况或危险因素的识别。筛检始于产前

筛检，例如对老年孕妇的唐氏综合症进行筛检，并持续一生。通常，建议对 49 岁以下的成年人每三年进行一次定期检查，对于 50 岁以上的成年人则建议每年进行一次检查。20-40 岁的成年人也应每 3-5 年进行一次心血管风险评估。年龄超过 40 岁且无危险因素的成年人，每年应进行高血压筛检[2,3]。

17-21 岁的成年人接受一次高脂血症筛检。此后，定期筛检从男性 35 岁开始，女性 45 岁开始[4]。对于患有高血压或高血脂症的成年人以及体重指数（BMI）大于 25 Kg / m2 的所有 40 岁以上的成年人，建议进行糖尿病筛检[5]。

老年人骨骼低矿物质密度（BMD）的患病率很高。建议对所有 65 岁以上的女性以及年龄在 65 岁以下，具有骨质疏松症危险因素的停经后女性进行筛检。包括具有低骨量，病史或骨折危险因素的临床表现的男性[6]。

筛检乳腺癌，肺癌和结直肠癌对老年人有效，因为临床试验指出，由于早期发现和更有效的治疗，被筛检病人的死亡率低于未筛检的死亡率[7,8]。

简单、快速的检查，例如血压测量和血液化学检查，是理想的筛检检查，因为该程序特别安全。筛检的不良反应包括筛检过程中的不适感，与筛检有关的风险，假阳性筛检结果（导致不必要的进一步检查和对患者的心理影响）以及过度诊断。但是，总的来说，大多数人都支持筛检。

改变生活方式，例如停止吸烟、健康饮食和规律运动，可以降低许多疾病的风险[9]。

药物预防是使用药物预防疾病，例如低剂量阿司匹林可以预防心血管疾病，钙或维生素 D 可以降低骨质疏松症的风险。

参考文献

1. Liang JL, Tiwari T, Moro P et al. Prevention of pertussis, tetanus and diphtheria with vaccines in the United States: Recommendations of the Advisory Committee on immunization practices (ACIP). MMWR Recomm Rep 2018;67:1
2. Ponka D. The periodic health examination in adults. CMAJ 2014;186:1245
3. Screening for high blood pressure in adults: US Preventive Services Task Force recommendation statement. Ann Intern Med 2015;163:1
4. 4. Strandberg TE, Kolehmainen L, Vuorio A. Evaluation and treatment of older patients with hypercholesterolemia: a clinical review. JAMA 2014;312:1136
5. Siu AL, US Preventive Services Task Force. Screening for abnormal blood glucose and type 2 diabetes mellitus: US Preventive Services Task Force Recommendation Statement. Ann Intern Med 2015;163:861
6. Gourlay ML, Fine JP, Preisser JS et al. Bone-density testing interval and transition to osteoporosis in older women. N Eng J Med 2012;366:225
7. Walter LC, Covinsky KE. Cancer screening in elderly patients: a framework for individualized decision making. JAMA 2001;285:2750
8. Snyder AH, Magnuson A, Westcott AM. Cancer screening in older adults. Med Clin North Am 2016;100:1101
9. Artand F, Dugravot A, Sabia S et al. Unhealthy lifestyle behaviors and disability in older adults: three-city cohort study. BMJ 2013;347:f4240

第二章

近期养生保健法

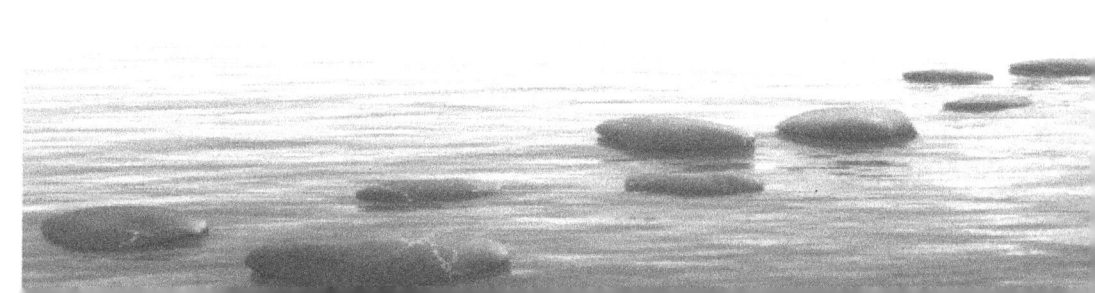

2.1 压力(stress)、双相剂量效应(hormesis)、平衡等稳性(homeostasis)

压力 (stress) 是任何物理,化学或生物因素(压力源,stressor)产生的刺激或信号组成的事件集合。这些刺激或信号激活体内的压力反应 (stress response) 或防卫机转 (fight or flight systems),从而释放因子于系统循环中以及局部中枢和周边组织内,用以抵消、适应和生存。[1]

人体在生活环境中会遇到各种压力。确实,压力是生活中无处不在的一部分。各种压力攻击包括热,辐射,缺氧,氧化压力,热量限制,植物化学物质,代谢,神经激素和蛋白毒性压力,环境毒素等。所有生物系统都具有内在反应能力,从而抵抗和适应外在及内在环境的条件。

有趣的是,压力的影响似乎是剂量依赖性的过程。轻度压力会诱导适应性的宿主防御机转,从而延长健康期 (healthspan) 和生命期 (lifespan),而过大的压力会引起有害影响,从而降低健康期和生命期。

这种现象被称为双相剂量效应(hormesis)，在生物体内和体外细胞培养研究中都已观察到。[2,3,4] 因此，压力可以对健康期和生命期产生正面或负面的影响。双相剂量效应被定义为对环境条件或因素的双相剂量反应，因此低剂量引起代偿或有益作用，而高剂量则对细胞或生物体产生失偿性或有害作用[5,6]。

一般而言，轻微、短暂和生理性的压力会激活多种生理系统，例如心血管，肌肉骨骼，神经内分泌和免疫系统，以增强人体保护或功能。这种压力适应性反应是大自然的基本生存机制之一，或称为自愈机能。但是，严重、持续和病理性的压力是失偿及适应不良的，并且已证明对健康期和生命期具有许多不利影响。[7]

Claude Bernard 在 1878 年首次指出，活生物体的生存构造部分存在于沐浴它们的流体中（内部因子或内部环境, internal milieu or internal environment），并且所有生理重要机制（生命）都依赖于稳定的内部环境或体内平衡等稳性 (homeostasis)。[8,9] 长期以来，人们一直认识到生物体维持自身稳定性的能力。身体健康与身体的「平衡」有关。正常健康生物体中大多数的生理指数，例如

血压，体温，血源性生理因子（例如氧气，葡萄糖，钠等）都保持在相对稳定的状态。这种稳定的内部因子(环境）被视为「平衡等稳性」(homeostasis)，即在一定范围内维持内部平衡条件。

压力是威胁到体内平衡等稳性的任何刺激。[10,11] 压力不仅指外部或内部环境对生物的压力挑战，还指生物体应对这些压力的反应。应对压力的生理反应是整个生物体内生物系统机转的协调调节，从而维持体内的平衡稳态或体内平衡等稳性。

所有活生物体都在为生存而不断奋斗，不仅要生存在环境压力下，还要生存在任何活动产生的生化和生理变化后果中。身体是一个自动适应系统，由于它具有适应能力，即使在适应不良的情况或疾病状态下，也可以保持生理稳定状态或体内平衡等稳性。简而言之，有益的压力 (hormetic stress；轻微、短暂和生理性的压力) 能够促进体内平衡等稳性及身体健康。

参考文献

1. Dhabhar FS, McEwen BS. Acute stress enhances while chronic stress suppresses immune function in vivo: a potential role for leukocyte trafficking. Brain Behav Immun 1997;11:286-306
2. Mattson MP. Hormesis defined. Ageing Res Rev 2008;7:1-7
3. Gems D, Partridge L. Stress-response hormesis and aging:"That which does not kill us makes us stronger". Cell Meta 2008;7:200-3
4. Rattan SIS. Hormesis in aging. Ageing Res Rev 2008;7:63-78
5. Calabresde EJ, Blain R. The occurrence of hermetic dose responses in the toxicological literature, the hormesis database: an overview. Toxicol Appl Pharmacol 2005;202:289-301
6. Mattson MP. Hormesis defined. Ageing Res Rev 2008;7:1-7
7. Dhabhar FS. The short-term stress response – Mother nature's mechanism for enhancing protection and performance under conditions of threat, challenge and opportunity. Frontiers Neuroendocrinology 2018;4:175-192
8. Bernard C. Les Phenomenes de la Vic. Paris 1878, two vols.
9. Cannon WR. Organization for physiological homeostasis. Physiol Rev 1929;9(3):399-431
10. Smith SM, Vale WW. The role of the hypothalamic-pituriary-adrenal axis in neuroendocrine responses to stress. Dial Clin Neurosci 2006;8:383-95
11. Pacak K, Palkovits M. Stressor specificity of central neuroendocrine responses: implications for stress- related disorders. Endocr Rev 2001;22:502-48

压力(stress)、双相剂量效应(hormesis)、平衡等稳性(homeostasis)

2.2 心脏优化

冠状动脉 (coronary arteries) 是心脏的血管。当冠状动脉部分或完全闭塞时，供应给心脏肌肉 (心肌、myocardium) 的血液减少或停止，就会分别发生心肌缺氧 (myocardial ischemia) 或心肌梗塞 (myocardial infarction)，分别导致心肌损伤或死亡。

冠心病 (亦称缺血性心脏病) 是心血管阻塞引起心肌缺氧所致。轻微、短暂及生理性的心肌缺氧会产生适应或代偿机转。反之严重、持续及病理性的心肌缺氧则会产生不适应或失偿机转。不论代偿或失偿机转都会激活神经内分泌系统、心脏重塑、及其他事件如：氧化作用、自噬作用 (细胞清除细胞废弃物的机转以维持细胞等穩性)、内皮细胞分泌的血管收缩素、一氧化氮、发炎诱发因子、生长因子等。

神经内分泌系统的激活主要是激活自主神经系统，及肾素-血管收缩素-醛固酮系统 (renin-angiotensin-aldosterone system)。轻微、短暂及生理性的交感神经系统激活，会增加心率，心收缩力及心输出量。但是严重、持续及病理性的交感神经系统

激活，却会对心脏细胞有不良作用，导致心脏功能丧失 [1,2,3]。生理性的肾素-血管收缩素-醛固酮 (renin-angiotensin-aldosterone) 系统激活，会导致血管收缩，细胞增生，醛固酮激素(aldosterone) 分泌，儿茶酚胺 (catecholamine) 的释出，从而维持短暂性的心血管系统等稳性 [4,5]。病理性的肾素-血管收缩素-醛固酮系统 (renin-angiotensin-aldosterone system) 激活会导致心脏、肾脏及其他器官纤维化，从而减少血管弹性，及增加心脏僵硬、不灵活 [4,5]。所以代偿性神经内分泌系统激活，会增加钠及水分保存，周边血管收缩，增加心收缩力，及激活对心脏恢复及重塑需要的诱发体，从而改善心输出量及心血管功能。

生理性或病理性的心肌缺氧会产生心脏重塑，会影响心脏细胞及心脏结构 [4]。代偿机转产生的心肌肥厚会减少心肌压力，从而改善及维持有效的心输出量及心血管功能 [6,7]。失偿机转产生的心脏重塑却会导致心室扩大、心肌肥厚、心脏纤维化及心血管功能恶化 [8]。

人体的新陈代谢会产生氧化反应物 (reactive oxygen species)，这些氧化反应物会影响心脏细胞内的蛋白质及讯息传导路径，包括调整心肌收缩功能的

蛋白质如：离子通道及心肌纤维蛋白质。并包括调整心肌细胞生长的讯息传导路径。心脏的氧化压力 (oxidative stress) 可能是因为抗氧化能力不足，或因为心脏负荷，神经内分泌系统激活，或发炎和免疫反应的介体 (例如 tumor necrosis factor, interleukin IL-1) 增加氧化反应物所致。心脏有过多的氧化反应物会导致收缩功能异常，激活心脏肥厚及凋亡（apoptosis，即程序性细胞死亡），调整纤维及胶原增加，及触发母组织金属蛋白酶 (matrix metalloproteinase，分解细胞外流液蛋白的酶) 增加[9]。

所以轻微、短暂，生理性的心肌缺氧是对心脏刺激压迫，会产生代偿机转，从而维持心血管系统等稳性及正常功能。而且是在分子，细胞，结构，组织及器官层面上。

心脏前准备作用 (ischemic preconditioning) 是于 1986 年 Murry 等[10]发现。短暂 (五分钟) 的心血管阻塞会在之后的心肌梗塞时减少心肌梗塞范围。我在大白鼠离体心脏亦观察到短暂 (五分钟) 的心肌缺氧会在之后心肌梗塞时减少心肌梗塞引起的心律不整及

收缩功能异常 (1986年未发表资料)。 文献已经建立心脏前准备作用是双相的现象：第一保护作用现象是在数分钟短暂的心肌缺氧后1至2小时产生；第二保护作用现象是在12至24小时后产生，且持续至3至4天[10,11,12]。 这二种保护作用现象是不同的，第一保护作用现象是已存在的蛋白质改变；第二保护作用现象是需要新的蛋白质合成。且第二保护作用现象产生的有利及保护作用与第一保护作用现象是相同有效[13]。

前准备作用已经在很多动物及临床实验中获得证实[10,14,15]。前准备作用可以保护之后的心肌梗塞引起的收缩功能异常[16]、心律不整[17,18]、凋亡（apoptosis，即程序性细胞死亡）[19]及心肌损伤[10,14,15]。轻微、短暂、生理性的心肌缺氧产生的前准备作用被公认为重大的心脏保护领域。

心脏前准备作用 (ischemic preconditioning) 是轻微的心肌缺氧，会在之后的心肌梗塞时减少心肌梗塞损伤。 心脏后准备作用 (ischemic postconditioning) 是在心肌梗塞期间轻微的心肌缺氧会减少心肌梗塞范围。 心脏间接准备作用 (remoteischemic preconditioning) 是于其他器官轻

微的缺氧产生心脏保护作用。这些心脏准备作用包括细胞膜受体的复杂讯号连锁反应，细胞内的酶激活及抑制粒线体（mitochondria）的凋亡讯号反应[20,21]。

心脏前准备作用可能自然而然地发生于人类。心肌梗塞前的心绞痛（pre-infarct angina）可能与心脏前准备作用相似。有心绞痛病史或心肌梗塞前有心绞痛的病人会有低死亡率，少发生心脏衰竭及休克[22]。这些心肌梗塞前心绞痛产生的有利及保护作用可能与心脏前准备作用有关。

心脏准备作用已成功地应用在冠心病患者。在进行心导管[23]或心脏手术[24]患者，心脏前准备作用能改善临床结果。在心肌梗塞患者，心脏后准备作用也能减少心肌梗塞范围及其他损伤[25-28]。

心脏间接准备作用常利用量血压时的血压带，打气到200mmHg五分钟及泄气五分钟，间歇地共三到五次[29]。在进行心导管或心脏手术病人，心脏间接准备作用亦可以减少心肌梗塞损伤及主要的心脏及脑血管有害事件[30-33]。此外，心脏间接前及后准备作用亦能有效地减少脑中风严重程度[34-38]。

药理准备作用 (模拟前准备作用) 是利用药物代替心肌缺氧来产生心脏保护作用。多种可能在心肌缺氧损伤机转作用的药物如：adenosine、nicorandil、erythropoietin、diazoxide、cyclosporine 等受试验评估。但是结果令人失望。目前认为心脏准备作用比药理准备作用较有效果 [20]。

心肌缺氧时产生很多的心脏保护作用讯号机转已被确认。这些讯号机转包括三个层面：诱发因子(triggers)、细胞内讯号连锁反应 (intracellular mediator cascade) 及作用器(effectors)。诱发因子如 adenosine、bradykinin、opioids 等分子，于心肌缺氧时自心脏细胞产生及释出。这些诱发因子激活细胞膜受体，产生细胞内蛋白激酶 (protein kinase) 的连锁反应，从而作用于作用器如粒线体 (mitochondria) 或细胞支架(cytoskeleton)，以稳定心脏细胞损伤及防备心脏细胞死亡 [20,21,33]。一氧化氮、蛋白激酶激活及粒线体是心脏准备作用产生的心脏保护机转重要要素 [20,21,34]。

因为安全及可行性，心脏准备作用是最能引发心脏保护的方法。心脏间接准备作用不需要直接操作

心血管，只需要利用量血压时的血压带，在上或下肢进行间歇性的打气及泄气[30-33]。运动是心脏保护的独立因子，运动也可减少心血管危险因素，如提高脂肪代谢，减重及增加胰岛素活性[39]。运动可引发心脏前准备作用，及在进行心导管手术患者减少心肌损伤[40]。一氧化氮(nitric oxide)是心脏前准备作用的诱发及作用因素[41-45]。静脉注射硝酸甘油(nitroglycerin)提升一氧化氮，可以在心肌缺氧时保护心脏[46]。

    扼要重述，轻微、短暂及生理性的心肌缺氧是对心脏刺激压迫，会产生代偿机转，从而维持心血管系统等稳性及正常功能，而且是在分子、细胞、结构、组织及器官层面上。经由此心脏便可得到心脏优化及保护作用。从而会在之后的严重、持续、病理性的心肌缺氧具有利及保护作用，减少不良心血管事件。所以心脏准备作用是最重要的养生保健法。因其可以预防最常见的也最致命的猝死、心肌梗塞及脑中风，最低限度可减少其发病率及死亡率。再者，健康的心血管系统分布及交互全身各系统。心脏准备作用不止保护心脏，也可保护其他器官如脑、肺、肾、肠、对缺氧及其他如毒物、休克、辐射剂等引起的损伤[47]。所以，文献证实人体具准备作用可能推动研发

能持续优化及保护心脏作用的模式或方法，最好能规律长期性保护心血管系统。人体能够募集各种适应性，代偿性机制，以反应各种刺激压迫而维持体内平衡等稳性和正常功能。 越来越明显的是，心脏优化和其他身体系统优化会启动代偿性适应，以维持心血管和身体的体内平衡等稳性，这是成功的抗老化策略的主要要点。

您可购买「养生血压计」(www.heartdisease.idv.tw) 实行心脏优化。

参考文献

1. Rundqvist, B., Elam, M., Bergmann-Sveroisdottivica, Y. et. al., 1997. Increased cardiac adrenergic drive precedes generalized sympathetic activation in human heart failure. Cir. 95(1),169-75.
2. Eichhorn, E.J., Bristow, M.R., 1996. Medical therapy can improve the biological properties of the chronically failing heart. A new era in the treatment of heart failure. Cir. 94(9),2285-96.
3. Mann, D.L., 1998. Basic mechanisms of disease progression in the failing heart: the role of excessive adrenergic drive. Prog. Cardiovasc. Ds.41(suppl),1-8.
4. Dell'Italia, L., Sabis, A., 2004. Activation of the rennin-angiotensin system in hypertrophy and heart failure. In Mann DL (ed):Heart failure: A companion to Baunwald's Heart Diseases. Philadelphia, Saunders;pp.129-143.
5. Schrier, R.W., Abraham, W.T., 1999. Hormones and hemodynamics in heart failure. N. Eng. J. Med. 341,577.
6. Cohn, J.N., Ferrari, R., Sharpe, N., 2000. Cardiac remodeling- concepts and clinical implications: a consensus paper from an international forum on cardiac remodeling. On behalf of an international Forum on cardiac remodeling. J. Am. Coll. Cardiol.35,569-82.
7. Swynghedauw, B., 1999. Molecular mechanism of myocardial remodeling. Physiol.Rev.79,215-62.
8. Pfeffer, M.A., Brauwald, E., 1990. Ventricular remodeling after myocardial infarction. Experimental observations and clinical implications. Cir.81,1161-72.
9. Grieve, D.J., Shah, A.M., 2003. Oxidative stress in heart failure. More than just damage. Eur. Heart J.24,2161
10. Murry, C.E., Jennings, R.B., Reimer, K.A., 1986. Preconditioning with ischemia: a delay of lethal cell injury

in ischemic myocardium. Cir. 74,1124-36.
11. Marber, M.S., Latchman, D.S., Walker, J.M., Yellon, D.M., 1993. Cardiac stress protein elevation 24 hours after brief ischemia or heat stress is associated with resistance to myocardial infarction. Cir.88,1264-72.
12. Kuzuya, T., Hoshida, S., Yamashita, N. et. al., 1993. Delayed effects of sublethal ischemia on the acquisition of tolerance to ischemia. Cir. Res.72,1293-9.
13. Shen, Y.T., Depre, C., Yan, L. et al., 2008. Repetitive ischemia by coronary stenosis induces a novel window of ischemic preconditioning. Cir.118,1961-9.
14. Sumeray, M.S., Yellon, D.M., 1998. Characterization and validation of a murine model of global ischemia-reperfusion injury. Mol. Cell.Biochem.186,61.
15. Schott, R.J., Rohmann, S., Braun, E.R., Schaper, W., 1990. Ischemic preconditioning reduces infarct size in swine myocardium. Cir. Res.66,1133
16. Cave, A.C., Hearse, D.J., 1991. Ischemic preconditioning and contractile function: studies with normothermic and hypothermic global ischemia. J. Mol.Cell. Cardiol.24,1113
17. Shiki, K., Hearse, D.J., 1987. Preconditioning of ischemic myocardium; reperfusion-induced arrhythmias. Am. J. Physiol.253,H1470
18. Vegh, A., Komori, S., Szekeres, L., Parratt, J.R., 1992. Antiarrhythmic effects of preconditioning in anesthetized dogs and rats. Cardiovas. Res. 26,487
19. Piot, C.A., Padmanaban, D., Ursell, P.C. et al., 1997. Ischemic preconditioning decreases apoptosis in rat hearts in vivo. Cir. 96,1598
20. Heusch, G., 2013. Cardioprotection: chances and challenges of its translation to the clinic. Lancet 381,166-75
21. Heusch, G., Boengler, K., Schulz, R., 2008. Cardioprotection: nitric oxide, protein kinases, and mitochondria. Cir. 118,1915-19.

22. Kloner, R.A., Shook, T., Przyklenk, K .et al., 1995. Previous angina alters in-hospital outcome in TIMI 4: a clinical correlate to preconditioning? Cir. 91,37-45
23. Leslay, W.K., Beach, D., 2003. Frequency and clinical significance of ischemic preconditioning during percutaneous coronary intervention. J. Am. Coll. Cardiol. 42,998-1003.
24. Walsh, S.R., Tang, T.Y., Kullar, P. et al., 2008. Ischemic preconditioning during cardiac surgery: systemic review and meta-analysis of perioperative outcomes in randomized clinical trials. Eur. J. Cardio. Thorac. Surg. 34,985-94.
25. Hansen, P.R., Thibault, H., Abdulla, J., 2010. Postconditioning during primary percutaneous coronary intervention: a review and meta-analysis. Int. J. Cardiol. 144,22-25.
26. Khan, A.R., Binabdulhak, A.A., Alastal, Y. et al., 2014. Cardioprotective role of ischemic postconditioning in acute myocardial infarction: a systemic review and meta-analysis. Am. Heart J. 168,512-21.
27. Staat, P., Rioufol, G., Piot, C. et al., 2005. Postconditioning the human heart. Cir. 112,2143-48.
28. Yang, X.C., Liu, Y., Wang, L.F. et al., 2007. Reduction in myocardial infarct size by postconditioning in patients after percutaneous coronary intervention. J. Invasive Cardiol. 19,424-30.
29. Heusch, G., Botker, H.E., Przyklenk, K. et al., 2015. Remote ischemic conditioning. J. Am. Coll. Cardiol. 65,177-95.
30. Thielmann, M., Kottenberg, E., Kleinbongard, P. et al., 2013 Cardioprotective and prognostic effects of remote ischemic preconditioning in patient undergoing coronary artery bypass surgery: a single-centre randomized, double-blind, controlled trial. Lancet 382,597-604.

31. Hode, S.P., Heck, P.M., Sharples, L. et al., 2009. Cardiac remote ischemic preconditioning in coronary stenting (CRISP stent) study: a prospective, randomized control trial. Cir. 119,820-7.
32. Davies, W.R., Brown, A.J., Watson, W. et al., 2013. Remote ischemic preconditioning improves outcome at 6 years after elective percutaneous coronary intervention: the CRISP stent trial long-term follow-up. Cir. Cardiovas. Interv. 6,246-51.
33. Crimi, G., Pica, S., Raineri, C. et al., 2013. Remote ischemic postconditioning of the lower limb during primary percutaneous coronary intervention safely reduces enzymatic infarct size in anterior myocardial infarction: a randomized controlled trial. J.A.C.C. Cardiovas. Interv. 6,1055-63.
34. Zhao, H., 2009. Ischemic postconditioning as a novel avenue to protect against brain injury after stroke. J. Cereb. Blood Flow Meta. 29,837-85.
35. Ren, C., Gao, M., Dorubos, D. et al., 2011. Remote ischemic postconditioning reduced brain damage in experimental ischemia/reperfusion injury. Neurol. Res. 33,514-9.
36. Hoda, M.N., Bhatia, K., Hafez, S.S. et al., 2014. Remote ischemic preconditioning is effective after embolic stroke in ovariectomized female mice. Transl. Stroke 5,484-90.
37. Hoda, M.N., Siddiqui, S., Herberg, S. et al., 2012. Remote ischemic conditioning is effective alone and in combination with intravenous tissue-type plasminogen activator in murine model of embolic stroke. Stroke 43,2794-99.
38. Ren, C., Wang, P., Wang, B. et al., 2015. Limb remote ischemic preconditioning in combination with postconditioning reduces brain damage and promotes neuroglobin expression in rat brain after ischemic stroke. Restor. Neurol. Neurosci. 33,369-79.

39. Fletcher, G.F., Blaire, S.N., Blumentahl, J, et al., 1992. Statement on exercise. Benefits and recommendations for physical activity programs for all Americans. A statement for health professionals by the Committee on exercise and cardiac rehabilitation of the Council on clinical Cardiology, Am Heart Ass. Cir. 86,340-44.
40. Lambiase, P.D., Edwards, R.J., Cusack, M.R. et al., 2003. Exercise-induced ischemia initiates the second window of protection in humans independent of collateral recruitment. J.A.C.C. 41,1174-82.
41. Bolli, R., Dawn, B., Tang, X.L. et al., 1998. The nitric oxide hypothesis of late preconditioning. Basic Res. Cardiol. 93,325-8.
42. Bolli, R., Bhatti, Z.A., Tang, X.L. et al., 1997. Evidence that late preconditioning against myocardial stunning in conscious rabbits is triggered by the generation of nitric oxide. Cir. Res. 81,42-52.
43. Qiu, Y., Rizvi, A., Tang, X.L. et al., 1997. Nitric oxide triggers late preconditioning against myocardial infarction in conscious rabbits. Am. J. Physio. 273,H2931-6.
44. Takano, H., Tang, X.L., Qiu, Y. et al., 1998. Nitric oxide donors induce late preconditioning against myocardial stunning and infarction in conscious rabbits via an antioxidant-sensitive mechanism. Cir. Re. 83,K73-84.
45. Banerjee, S., Tang, X.L., Qiu, Y. et al., 1999. Nitroglycerin induces late preconditioning against myocardial stunning via a protein kinase C dependent pathway. Am. J .Physiol. 277,H2488-94.
46. Leesar, M.A., Stoddard, M.F., Dawn, B. et al., 2001. Delayed preconditioning-mimetic action of nitroglycerin in patients undergoing coronary angioplasty. Cir 103,2935-41.
47. Przyklenk, K., Whittaker, P., 2011. Remote ischemic preconditioning: current knowledge, unresolved questions, and future priorities. J. Cardiovas. Pharmacol. Ther. 16(3-4), 255-9.

2.3 肺优化

相对来说，对肺而言，对等或类似心血管，心血管阻塞，及心肌缺氧便是气管、气管阻塞(支气管收缩或痉挛)、及通气障碍。

肺的主要功能是气体交换。气管是空气进出肺部做气体交换的管道。呼吸症状大部分是因为气管阻塞引起气流阻力增加。气喘（asthma）是一种肺病，其特征是间歇地短暂性的气管肌肉收缩，气管狭窄及阻塞，从而明显的增加气流阻力。气喘病的基本病变是因过敏，病毒感染，及对环境因素敏感引起气管慢性发炎。此潜在的发炎会引起气管肌肉过度反应。运动（特别是寒冷干燥天气）或接触吸菸、环境污染、病毒、过敏原时，通常会释出气管收缩化学物质及其他潜在性的诱发因子，从而引起强劲的气管收缩。

气管收缩（bronchospasm）包括导致气管狭窄的收缩素如 leukotrienes, histamine, endothelin 1, bradykinin 等[1]，发炎反应如水肿、发炎诱发因子、黏液分泌[2,3]及气管重塑(airway remodeling)如气管变厚、纤维化、肺弹性下降、气管结构改变等[4,5,6]。

气管重塑 (airway remodeling) 是指气管壁细胞和分子成分数量或结构的变化。它包括气管上皮细胞的损伤，黏液分泌细胞 (goblet cell) 增生，黏液腺增大及黏液分泌增多；气管下皮细胞转变则包括纤维细胞增生及激活；细胞外组织液蛋白沉淀及调整改变，血管增生及血管重塑，气管肌肉增生及肥厚。这些转变会导致气管壁变厚，气管狭窄及气流限制引起不太会逆转的气管阻塞 [4,5,6]。

运动诱发气管收缩（exercise-induced bronchospasm）包括运动中或后产生的气管狭窄，导致的呼吸症状如气喘、胸闷、咳嗽、呼吸困难及喘鸣（wheezing）等 [7]。运动诱发气管收缩可出现在正常人或气喘病人。运动诱发气管收缩反应已有很好描述，包括其生理转变取决于运动量及持续期间。少于 4 分钟的运动不会产生运动诱发气管收缩反应，而持续运动 8、12 或 16 分钟会产生典型的运动诱发气管收缩反应，及于 30 至 60 分钟后慢慢恢复 [8,9]。此外，在经过之前运动诱发气管收缩反应后 60 分钟内重复运动则会产生比前一次更轻微及短暂的气管收缩。这不反应期是气管收缩事件前的「暖身」（warm-up）或「闪过、避开」（running through）现象，对气

管是有利及保护作用的 [9,10,11]。这准备作用类似心脏前准备作用，即于事件前轻微及短暂约 16 分钟的运动会优化保护气管，从而在 60 分钟内的持续运动会出现较轻微的气管收缩反应。所以尽管运动能诱发气管收缩，很多证据指出规律运动及有氧运动准备作用，能减少运动诱发气管收缩的频繁及严重度。动物实验证实有氧运动训练可有效减少气管发炎，发炎细胞渗透，氧化压力及气管重塑，气管水肿等。人体实验亦证实有氧运动训练可有效改善气喘症状频率及严重度，心肺功能健康及肺功能正常 [12]。所以，能诱发气管收缩至无反应期的运动模式是对气管有利的，可导致肺优化及保护作用。

运动后产生「暖身」或「闪过、避开」气管收缩不反应期的机转包括血液高浓度 catecholamines，发炎细胞诱发因子 (mast cell mediators) 减少，神经胜肽 (neuropeptides) 释出减少，气管肌肉反应减少，气管保护作用诱发因子如 prostaglandin 释出，及诱发气管收缩的受体敏感度或调节度减少 [13]。

另一方面，心脏间接准备作用是于心脏血管组织或器官进行轻微短暂的缺血再灌流现象，能对其他

组织及器官产生保护作用。

本来发现可保护心脏，之后再发现心脏间接准备作用亦能保护其他非心脏的组织及器官如肾、肺、肝、肠、胃等[14]。

心脏前准备作用及药理前准备作用研究指出可减轻肺部损伤[15,16]。心脏间接准备作用亦能减轻因出血性休克而产生的肺损伤[17]。

心脏后准备作用能改善肺部缺血再灌流时产生的病理转变及改善肺的氧合作用[18]。经过心脏间接准备作用后，健康成人进行低氧运动会减低肺动脉压和改善通气效能及气流交换[19]。

心脏间接准备作用能减少肺部发炎及发炎细胞积聚[20]。很多外科手术如心脏手术、骨手术、肺切除术、肺移植手术等，会产生急性肺损伤及肺功能异常。这些都是主要引起发病率及死亡的原因。心脏间接准备作用能减少此等不良后果[21-25]。

总而言之，规律运动及有氧运动准备作用，及心脏间接准备作用都可以优化和保护气管及肺部。在之后的持续运动或缺血再灌流时会产生有利及保护作用。这准备作用现象可能推动研发能维持肺部持续优化及保护状态的模式或方法，最好是规律性及长期性的保护呼吸系统。

参考文献

1. Wen AR, Syyong HT, Siddiqui S et al. Airway contractility and remodeling: Links to asthma symptoms. Pulm Pharmacol Therap 2013;26:3-12.
2. Elwood W, Barnes PJ, Chung KF. Airway hyperresponsiveness is associated with inflammatory cell infiltration in allergic brown Norway rats. Int Arch Allergy Immunol 1992;99(1):91-7.
3. Elwood D W, Lotvall JO, Barnes PJ et al. Characterization of allergen-induced bronchial hyperresponsiveness and airway inflammation in actively sensitized brown Norway rats. J Allergy Clin Immunol 1991;88(6):951-60.
4. McAnnldty RJ. Models and approaches to understand the role of airway remodeling in disease. Pulm Pharmacol Therap 2011;24:478-86.
5. Rydell-Tormanen K, Risse PA, Kauabar V, Bagchi R, Czubryt MP, Johnson JR. Smooth muscle in tissue remodeling and hyperreactivity: Airway and arteries. Pulm Pharmacol Therap 2013;26:13-23.
6. Ward C, Pais M, Bish R et al. Airway inflammation, basement membrane thickening and bronchial hyperresponsiveness in asthma. Thorax 2002;57(4):309-16.
7. Weilu JM, Bonini S, Coifman R et al. American Academy of allergy, asthma and immunology work group report: exercise-induced asthma. J Allergy Clin Immunol 2007;119:1349-58.
8. Silverman M, Anderson SD. Standardization of exercise tests in asthmatic children. Arch Dis Child 1972;47:882-9.
9. Weiler-Ravell D, Godfrey S. Do exercise- and antigen-induced asthma utilize the same pathways? Antigen provocation in patients rendered refractory to exercise-induced asthma. J Allergy Clin Immunol 1981;67:391-7.

10. Reiff DB, Choudry NB, Pride NB et al. The effect of prolonged submaximal warm-up exercise on exercise-induced asthma. Am Rev Respir Dis 1989;139:479-84.
11. McKenzie DC, McLuckie SL, Stirling DR. The protective effects of continuous and interval exercise in athletes with exercise-induced asthma. Med Sci Sports Exerc 1994;26:951-6.
12. Craig TJ and Dispenza MC. Benefits of exercise in asthma. Ann Allergy Asthma Immunol 2013;110:133-40.
13. Larsson J, Anderson SD, Dahlen SE, Dahlen B. Refractoriness to exercise challenge: A review of the mechanisms old and new. Immunol Allergy Clin N Am 2013;33:329-345.
14. Candilio L, Malik A, Hausenloy DJ. Protection of organs other than the heart by remote ischemic conditioning. J Cardiovas Med 2013;14:193-205.
15. Turan NN, Demiryurek AT. Preconditioning effects of peroxynitrite in the rat lung. Pharmacol Res 2006;54:380-8.
16. Yildiz G, Demiryurek AT, Gumusel B et al. Ischemic preconditioning modulates ischemia-reperfusion injury in the rat lung: role of adenosine receptors. Eur J Pharamacol 2007;556:144-50.
17. Jan WC, Chen CH, Tsai PS, Huang CJ. Limb ischemic preconditioning mitigates lung injury induced by hemorrhagic shock/resuscitation in rats. Resuscitation 2011;82:760-6.
18. Xia ZY, Gao J, Ancharaz AK et al. Ischemic postconditioning protects lung from ischemia-reperfusion injury by up-regulation of heme-oxygenase 1. Injury. Int J Care Injured 2010;41:510-6.
19. Kim CH, Sajgalik P, ItersonEHV, Jae SY, Johnson BD. The effect of remote ischemic preconditioning on pulmonary vascular pressure and gas exchange in healthy humans during hypoxia. Resp Physiol Neurobiology 2019;161:62-6.
20. Peralta C, Fermandez L, Panes J et. al. Preconditioning

protects against systemic disorders associated with hepatic ischemia-reperfusion through blockade of tumor necrosis factor-induced P-selectin up-regulation in the rat. Hepatology 2001;33:100-113.
21. Harkin DW, Barros D'Sa AA, McCallion K et al. Ischemic preconditioning before lower limb ischemia-reperfusion protects against acute lung injury. J Vasc Surg 2002;35:1264-73.
22. Kharbanda RK, Li J, Konstantinov IE et al. Remote ischemic preconditioning protects against cardiopulmonary bypass-induced tissue injury: a preclinical study. Heart 2006;92:1506-11.
23. Li G, Chen S, Lu E, Luo W. Cardiac ischemic preconditioning improves lung preservation in valve replacement operations. Ann Thorac Surg 2001;71:631-5.
24. Cheung MM, Kharbanda RK, Konstantinov IE et al. Randomized controlled trial of the effects of remote ischemic preconditioning on children undergoing cardiac surgery: first clinical application in humans. J Am Coll Cardiol 2006;47:2277-82.
25. Zhou W, Zeng D, Chen R et al. Limb ischemic preconditioning reduces heart and lung injury after an open heart operation in infants. Pediatr Cardiol 2010;31:22-29.

2.4 肠优化

现代人类典型的每日三餐饮食，会导致饮食过量及代谢疾病，特别是加上缺乏运动。节食 (热量限制，calorie restriction) 是减少热量的摄取，但是须充分营养的饮食方式，能延长动物及人类的健康期及生命期[1]。禁食 (fasting) 能改善疾病指数，减少氧化刺激作用及维持学习及记忆功能。在禁食期间中，让细胞受轻微刺激，而细胞会适应地应对这些轻微刺激来抑制疾病[1]。

节食通常是每天减少 10%至 30%热量饮食[2]。间歇性断食 (intermittent fasting) 则是每周一至两天相当多的热量限制 (75%-90%的饮食量)[3]。节食及间歇性断食同样有效。节食加上间歇性断食常被应用而产生更大效应[1]。

至目前为止，仍未有随机临床试验决定节食及间歇性断食的效应，但是伊斯兰教信徒 (穆斯林) 在斋月里执行的一个月斋戒后会改善胰岛素敏感度，血糖及血脂控制[4,5,6]。

节食可有效减重、血脂、血压、血糖及血液细胞量[7]。节食加上间歇性断食可减体重，体脂肪，及缺血性心脏病风险[8]。

间歇性断食可增加生命期[9]，减少癌病及心血管疾病死亡率[10]，改善胰岛素敏感度[11]，减少氧化压力[12]，发炎[12]，及减少疾病如糖尿病和心血管疾病的风险[13]。

动物实验指出，间歇性断食对很多健康指标具极大有益作用，及对抗疾病如糖尿病，心血管疾病，癌及神经疾病如阿兹海默氏病(老年痴呆)，巴金森氏病及脑中风。临床试验指出，间歇性断食能改善很多健康指标，包括胰岛素耐受性及减少心血管疾病危险因子。

动物实验亦指出，间歇性节食能减重及增加生命期[14]，减少血脂肪，体脂肪及保持身材精瘦[15]，改善糖代谢(减少血糖及胰岛素量)及脂肪酸代谢[16]，增加胰岛素敏感度及改善血糖耐受性[15]，影响荷尔蒙[17,18]，减少基本心跳及血压及加强心血管代偿机转[17]，改善脑功能[19]。

间歇性节食可预防及治疗糖尿病[20]；间歇性节食逆转糖尿病的细胞及分子作用机转包括增加胰岛素受体讯号敏感度[21]及改变其他讯号通道如改善粒线体功能，激活粒线体产生及自噬机转(细胞清除细胞废弃物的机转以维持细胞等穩性)等[22,23,24]。

间歇性断食有极大心脏保护作用，能减少心肌梗塞损伤范围，及改善生存率及恢复心脏功能[25,26,27]。亦可减低血压[28]，增加心率变度(以控制心率)[29]，减少胰岛素耐受度[20,28]及血中胆固醇及三甘油脂[30,31]。

亦有报告间歇性断食可改善神经系统创伤[32,33]，脊髓创伤[32,33]，周边神经病变[34]，降低脑中风后的大脑损伤和功能丧失[35,36]，改善阿兹海默氏病(老年痴呆)，帕金森氏病[37]，及改善很多癌症的病情[38]。

临床试验指出，节食能减轻血管硬化[39]及改善肾功能[40]。间歇性断食可减体重及新陈代谢危险因子[41,42]，减少胰岛素耐受性[43]，减少心血管疾病[44]及癌症危险因子[45]。

伊斯兰教自 1443 年前起是第一个及唯一有执行节食及间歇性断食的修行宗教。这宗教常规比 McCay 等[46]于 1935 年发现的节食早了一千多年。全世界的穆斯林执行着每年一度的斋月 (回历 Ramadan) 一个月的节食并或不并全年每星期兩天的间歇性断食修行 (免除严重病人、儿童、经期及哺乳期妇女执行)。所谓斋月是伊斯兰历每年的第九个月份，是伊斯兰信仰中非常神圣的一个修行月份。在这个斋戒月里，数以亿计的穆斯林，每天自黎明至日落期间断食。斋月节食可提升有益胆固醇 (高密度脂蛋白，high-density lipoprotein cholesterol，"good" cholesterol，HDL)。减少坏胆固醇 (低密度脂蛋白，low-density lipoprotein cholesterol，"bad" cholesterol，LDL)[47,48]，斋月节食可减轻体重，体脂肪及体重指数[49]，及改善胰岛素敏感度。斋月节食可降低血压[47,48,49,50]，抵抗系统性发炎及氧化压力[51]引起的慢性疾病如癌症及心血管疾病[52]。

节食及间歇性断食对生理功能产生复相作用，即在低程度时产生有利作用，但在高程度时则会产生有害作用。所以节食及间歇性断食的程度及时间决定其产生有利或有害作用[53]。至目前为止，节食及间歇

性断食的方法仍是随意的。每年一个月节食并或不并每周两日的间歇性断食是安全，方便，容易适应及遵守的，因为以亿而计的穆斯林已经执行了逾1443年，尚未发生有害作用。

节食及间歇性断食的作用机转包括提高细胞代偿或防御机转[54,55]，重塑[56]，减少氧化压力，粒线体异常，发炎，调节凋亡（apoptosis，即程序性细胞死亡）及自噬功能[57]。

自噬功能或称自体吞噬(autophagy，self-eating)是细胞溶酶体(lysosome)分解过程及保护机转，用以淘汰受损细胞内小胞器(organelles)，滞留无用的蛋白质及入侵的病原体，从而维持细胞及组织等稳性(homeostasis)及预防很多病症如糖尿病、高血压、肝病、癌症、神经疾病、自主免疫疾病及感染等。肠道是一器官系统，其生理目标是吸收养分。节食及间歇性断食是对肠道的养分刺激压力，能产生细胞防御或代偿机转及自噬功能，所以对细胞等稳性及正常功能扮演着重要角色，从而对健康及肌肉、肝、胆、肾、心脏、神经系统等器官系统产生准备及保护作用[58]。

另一方面，以前的研究指出前准备作用能对很多器官系统如神经、心脏、肝胆肠道、肾及肌肉等系统产生保护作用[59,60]。胃黏膜的短暂缺氧可保护之后持续的缺氧再灌流产生的胃黏膜损伤。这指出肠道亦有前准备保护作用[61]。在兔子实验中，心脏间接前准备作用能保护肠道收缩功能[62]。大白鼠进行小肠移植手术前，心脏前准备间接作用能保护手术引起的肠道缺氧损伤[63]。Brozozowski 等报告心脏前准备间接作用可以保护胃的缺氧损伤[64]。利用经前准备作用后病人的血液，Zitta 等报告它可以保护病人肠道细胞对缺氧的损伤[65]。心脏间接准备作用亦可拯救因肠道血管阻塞引起的肠道损伤。这有利的保护作用与肠道发炎减少及肠道新生细胞增加有关[66]。再者，心血管手术前会造成肠道损伤是因为手术相关因素，造成肠道血流量减少，Li 等指出在进行心血管手术患者，心脏间接准备作用可保护肠道的功能[67]。

扼要重述：经节食/间歇性断食及前准备作用，肠道便可得到刺激、优化及保护作用，从而产生很多有利效果。这准备作用现象可能推动研发维持肠道持续优化及保护状态的模式或方法，最好是规律性及长期性的保护肠道系统。

参考文献

1. Most J, Tosti V, Redman LM, Fontana L. Calorie restriction in humans: an update. Aging Res Reviews 2017;39:36-45.
2. Lee SH, Min KJ. Calorie restriction and its mimetics. BMBRep 2013;86(1):7-13.
3. Bernosky AR et al. Intermittent fasting vs daily calorie restriction for type 2 diabetes prevention: a review of human findings. Transl Res 2014;June 12(Epubahead of print).
4. Shariatpanshi ZV et al. Effect of Ramadan fasting on some indices of insulin resistance and components of the metabolic syndrome in healthy male adults. Br J Nutr 2008;100(1):147-51.
5. Al-Shafei AI. Ramadan fasting ameliorates oxidative stress and improves glycemic control and lipid profile in diabetic patients. Eur J Nutr 2014 Jan 19(Epubahead of print).
6. Shehab A et al. Favorable changes in lipid profile: the effects of fasting after Ramadan. PLoS One 2012;7(10):e47615.
7. Walford RL, Weber L, Panor S. Calorie restriction and aging as viewed from biosphere 2. Receptor 1995;5(1):29-33.
8. Klempel MC et al. Intermittent fasting combined with calorie restriction is effective for weight loss and cardio-protection in obese women. Nutr J 2012;11:98.
9. Mattson MP, Wan R. Beneficial effects of intermittent fasting and calorie restriction on the cardiovascular and cerebrovascular systems. J Nutr Biochem 2005;16(3):129-37.
10. Buschomyer WC et al. Effect of intermittent fasting with

or without calorie restriction on prostate cancer5 growth and survival in SCID mice. Prostate 2010;70(10):1037-43.
11. Lu J et al. Alternate day fasting impacts the brain insulin-signaling pathway of young adult male C57BL/6 mice. J Neurochem 2011;117(1):154-63.
12. Castello L et al. Alternate-day fasting protects the rat heart against age-induced inflammation and fibrosis by inhibiting oxidate damage and NF-KB activation. Free Raic Biol Med 2010;48(1):47-54.
13. Wan R, Camandola S, Mattson MP. Intermittent food deprivation improves cardiovascular and neuroendocrine responses to stress in rats. J Nutri 2003;133(6):1921-9.
14. Goodrick CL, Ingram OK, Reynolds MA, Freeman JR, Cider NL. Effects of intermittent fasting upon growth and life span in rats. Gerontology 1982;28:233-41
15. Gotthardt JD, Verpent JL, Yeomans BL, Yang JA, Yasrebi A, Roepke TA, Bello NT. Intermittent fasting promotes fat loss with lean mass retention, increased hypothalamic norepinephrine content, and increased neuropeptide Y gene expression in diet-induced obese male mice. Endocrinology 2016;157:679-91.
16. Anson RM. Guo Z, de'Cabo R et al. Intermittent fasting dissociates beneficial effects of dietary restriction on glucose metabolism and neuronal resistance to injury from calorie intake. Proc Natl Acad Sci USA 2003;100:6216-6220.
17. Wan R, Camandola S, Mattson MP. Intermittent fasting deprivation improves cardiovascular and neuroendocrine responses to stress in rats. J Nutr 2003;133:1921-9.
18. Martin B, Pearson M, Brenneman R et al. Gonadal transcriptome alterations in response to dietary energy intake: sensing the reproductive environment. PLoS One 2009;4(1):e4146.
19. Li L, Wang Z, Zuo Z. Chronic intermittent fasting improves cognitive functions and brain structures in mice.

PLoS One 2013;8(6):e66069.
20. Belkacemi L, Selselet-Attou G, Louchami K, Sener A, Malaisse WJ. Intermittent fasting modulation of the diabetic syndrome in sand rats :LII. In vivo investigations. Int J Mol Med 2010;26:759-65.
21. Sequea DA, Sharma N, Arias EB, Cartee GD. Calorie restriction enhances insulin-stimulated glucose uptake and Akt phosphorylation in both fast-twitch and slow-twitch skeletal muscle of 24-month-old rats. J Gerontol A Biol Sci Med Sci 2012;67:1279-85.
22. Descamps O, Riondel J, Ducros V, Roussel A<. Mitochondrial production of reactive oxygen species and incidence of age-associated lymphoma in OF1 mice: effect of alternate day fasting. Mech Ageing Dev 2005;126:1185-91.
23. Cheng A, Yang Y, Zhou Y et al. Mitochondrial SIRT3 mediates adaptive responses of neurons to exercise and metabolic and excitatory challenges. Cell Metab 2016;23:128-42.
24. Longo VD, Mattson MP. Fasting: molecular mechanisms and clinical application. Cell Metab 2014;19:181-92.
25. Ahmet I, Wan R, Mattson MP, Lakatta EG, Talan M. Cardioprotection by intermittent fasting in rats. Cir 2005;112:3115-21.
26. Godar RJ, Ma X, Liu H et al. Repetitive stimulation of autophagy-lysosome machinery by intermittent fasting preconditions the myocardium to ischemia-reperfusion injury. Autophagy 2015;11:1537-60.
27. Katare RG, Kakinuma Y, Arikwa M, Yamasaki F, Sato T. Chronic intermittent fasting improves the survival following large myocardial ischemia by activation of BDNF/VEGF/D13K signaling pathway. J Mol Cell Cardiol 2009;46:405-12.
28. Wan R, Camandola S, Mattson MP. Intermittent food deprivation improves cardiovascular and neuroendocrine

responses to stress in rats. J Nutr 2003;133:1921-9.
29. Mager DE, Wan R, Brown M et al. Calorie restriction and intermittent fasting alter spectral measures of heart rate and blood pressure variability in rats. FASEB 2006;20:631-7.
30. Varady KA, Roohk DJ, Loe YC, McEvoy-Hein BK, Hellersteir MK. Effects of modified alternate-day fasting regimens on adipocyte size, triglyceride metabolism, and plasma adiponectin levels in mice. J Lipid Res 2007;48:2212-9.
31. Belkacemi L, Selselet-Atton G, Hupkens E et al. Intermittent fasting modulation of the diabetic syndrome in streptozotocin-injected rats. Int J Endocrinol 2012;962012.
32. Plunet WT, Lam CK, Lee JH, Liu J, Telzlaff W. Prophylactic dietary restriction may promote functional recovery and increase lifespan after spinal cord injury. Ann NY Acad Sci 2010;1198(suppl 1):E1-11.
33. Jeong MA, Plunet W, Streijger F et.al. Intermittent fasting improves functional recovery after rat thoracic contusion spinal cord injury. J Neurotrauma 2011;28:479-92.
34. Madorsky I, Opalach K, Waber A et al. Intermittent fasting alleviates the neuropathic phenotype in a mouse model of Charcot-Marie-Tooth disease. Neurobiol Dis 2009;34:146-54.
35. Yu ZF, Mattson MP. Dietary restriction and 2-deoxyglucose administration reduce focal ischemic brain damage and improve behavioral outcome: evidence for a preconditioning mechanism. J Neurosci Res 1999;57:830-9.
36. Arumugam TV, OPhillips TM, Cheng A et al. Age and energy intake interact to modify cell stress pathways and stroke outcome. Ann Neurol 2010;67:41-52.
37. Mattson MP. Energy intake and exercise as determinants of brain health and vulnerability to injury and disease. Cell Meta 2012;16:706-22.

38. Lee C, Raffaghello L, Brandhorst S, Safdie FM et al. Fasting cycles retard growth of tumors and sensitize a range of cancer cell types to chemotherapy. Sci Transl Med 2012;4,124 ral 27.
39. Fontana L, Meyer TE, Klein S, Holloszy JO. Long-term calorie restriction is highly effective in reducing the risk for atherosclerosis in humans. Proc Natl Acad Sci USA 2004;101:6659-63.
40. Giordani I, Malandrucco I, Donno S et al. Acute caloric restriction improves glomerular filtration rate in patients with morbid obesity and type 2 diabetes. Diabetes Meta 2014;40:158-60.
41. Anastasion CA, Karfopoulou E, Yannakoulia M. Weight regaining: from statistics and behaviors to physiology and metabolism. Metabolism 2015;64:1395-1407.
42. Johnson JB, Summer W, Cutler RG et al. Alternate day calorie restriction improves clinical findings and reduces markers of oxidative stress and inflammation in overweight adults with moderate asthma. Free Radic Biol Med 2007;42:665-74.
43. Harrie M, Wright C, Pegington M et al. The effect of intermittent energy and carbohydrate restriction and daily energy restriction on weight loss and metabolic disease risk markers in overweight women. Br J Nutr 2013;1-14.
44. Mattson MP, Longo VD, Harvie M. Impact of intermittent fasting on health and disease processes. Aging Res Reviews 2017;39:46-58.
45. Hursting SD, DiGiovanni J, Danneuberg AJ et al. Obesity, energy balance and cancer: new opportunities for prevention. Cancer Prev Res 2012;5:1260-72.
46. McCay CM, Crowell MF, Marnard LA. The effect of retarded growth upon the length of life span and upon the ultimate body size. J Nutr 1935;10:63-79.
47. Rahman M, Rashid M, Basher S et al. Improved serum HDL cholesterol profile among Bangladeshi male students

during Ramadan fasting. East Mediterr Health J 2004;10(1-2):131-7.
48. Nematy M, Alnezhad-Namaghi M et. al. Effects of Ramadan fasting on cardiovascular risk factors: a prospective observational study. Nutr J 2012;11:69.
49. Ziaee V, Razaei M, Ahmadinejad Z et. al. The changes of metabolic profile and weight during Ramadan fasting. Singapore Med J 2006;47(5):409
50. Shariatpanahi ZV, Shariatpanahi MV, Shahbazi S, Hossaini A, Abadi A. Effects of Ramadan fasting on some indices of insulin resistance and components of the metabolic syndrome in healthy male adults. Br J Nutr 2008;100:147-51.
51. Faris MAE, Jahrami HA, Obaideen NA, Madkour MI. Impact of diurnal intermittent fasting during Ramadan on inflammatory and oxidative stress markers in healthy people: systemic review and metaanalysis. J Nutr Intermediary Meta 2019;15:18-26.
52. Weiss EP, Fontana L. Calorie restriction: powerful protection for the aging heart and vasculature. Am J Phsiol Heart Cir Physiol 2011;301:H1205-19.
53. Li X, Yang T, Sun Z. Hormesis in health and chronic diseases. Trends Endocrinol Meta 2019;30(12):944-58.
54. Aly KB, Piplciu JL, Hinson WG et al. Chronic calorie restriction induces stress proteins in the hypothalamus of rats. Mech Ageing Dev 1994;76:11-23.
55. Ehrenfried JA, Evers BM, Chu KV, Townsend CM, Thompson JC. Calorie restriction increases the expression of heat shock protein in the gut. Ann Surg 1996;223:592-7.
56. Doy Y, Grepersen S, Ahao J et al. Morphometric and biomechanical intestinal remodeling induced by fasting in rats. Digestive Ds Sci 2002;47(5):1158-68.
57. Marzetti E, Wholgemuth SE, Anton SD et al. Cellular mechanisms of cardioprotection by calorie restriction: state of the science and future perspectives. Clin Geriatr

Med 2009;25:715-32.
58. Bagherniya M, Butler AE, Barreto GE, Sahebkar A. The effect of fasting or calorie restriction on autophagy induction: A review. Ageing Res Reviews 2018;47:183-97.
59. Peralta C, Prats N, Xaus C, Gelpi E, Rosello-Catafau J. Protective effect of liver ischemia preconditioning on liver and lung injury induced by hepatic ischemia-reperfusion in the rat. Hepatology 1999;30:1481-9.
60. Candilio L, Malik A, Hausenloy DJ. Protection of organs other than the heart by remote ischemic conditioning. J Cardiovasc Med 2013;14:193-205.
61. Pajdo R, Closa D, Xaus C et al. Ischemic preconditioning, the most effective gastroprotective intervention: involvement of prostaglandins, nitric oxide, adenosine and sensory nerves. Eur J Pharmacol 2001;427:263-76.
62. Dickson EW, Tubbs RJ, Porcaro WA et al. Myocardial preconditioning factors evoke mesenteric ischemic tolerance via opioid receptors and K(ATP) channels. Am J Physiol Heart Cir Physiol 2002;283:H22-8.
63. Saeki I, Matsuura T, Hayashida M, Taguchi T. Ischemic preconditioning and remote ischemic preconditioning have protective effect against cold ischemia-reperfusion injury of rat small intestine. Pediatr Surg Int 2011;27:857-62.
64. Brzozowski T, Konturek PC, Pajdo R et al. Importance of brain-gut axis in the gastroprotection induced by gastric and remote preconditioning. J Physiol Pharmacol 2004;55:165-77.
65. Zitta K, Meybohm P, Bein B et al. Serum from patients undergoing remote ischemic preconditioning protects cultured human intestinal cells from hypoxia induced damage: involvement of matrix metalloproteinase 2 and 9. Mol Med 2012;18:29-37.
66. Zhu H, Bindi E, Lee CM et al. Remote ischemic conditioning: a novel treatment strategy to minimize the

intestinal damage of midgut volvulus. J Am Coll Surg 2019;229(4 suppl 1):S216.
67. Li C, Li YS, Xu M et al. Limb remote ischemic preconditioning for intestinal and pulmonary protection during elective open infrarenal abdominal aortic aneurysm repair randomized controlled trial. J Am Soc Anesthesiol 2013;118:842-52.

2.5 全身优化

人体有十个器官系统，其组成部分及功能如下：

	系统名称	主要器官或组织	功能
1	神经系统	大脑、脊髓周边神经及神经节、感觉器官	控制及调整很多人体机能、意识状况、认知
2	心血管系统	心脏、血管、血液	人体血液运输
3	呼吸系统	鼻、咽、喉、气管、支气管、肺	氧气及二氧化碳交换
4	肠道系统	口、咽、食道、胃、肠道、肺、肝、胆囊	营养、矿物质及水分的消化和吸收
5	泌尿系统	肾、输尿管、膀胱、尿道	矿物质、水份及废物的排除，以控制血液黏稠度
6	肌肉骨骼系统	软骨、骨骼、韧带、腱、关节、肌肉	人体支撑、保护、及走动、产生红血球
7	免疫系统	白血球、淋巴管、淋巴结、脾脏、胸腺	防卫外来病原体的侵入

8	内分泌系统	分泌贺尔蒙的腺体或细胞	控制及调整很多人体机能如：生长、新陈代谢、电解质平衡等
9	生殖系统	性器官	生殖
10	皮肤系统	皮肤	保护创伤、防御外来侵入病原、调整体温

　　与前述心脏、肺、及肠道准备作用相似，我们同样可以刺激、优化及保护所有人体十个器官系统。这准备作用现象可能推动研发能维持全身持续优化及保护状态的模式或方法，最好是规律性及长期性的保护全身器官系统。 因为器官或组织缺血/再灌流损伤是全球最常见的罹病率及死亡率原因。 全身器官系统准备作用是最重要的养生保健法，因为可以预防疾病，甚至是最常见又致命的疾病如：猝死、心肌梗塞及脑中风，至少可以减少罹病及死亡率。 如果您没病，便是健康。 如果您受病痛所苦，或死于致命的疾病，那么您肯定是不健康。

　　间接准备作用通常是利用量血压时所用的血压带，打气5分钟及泄气5分钟，间歇共3至5次。但这是随意选择，最佳模式或方法仍未有确认。 再者，

有否其他更好或最佳能诱发准备及保护作用的模式或方法?

注意缺氧或准备作用所需程度，及第二保护作用现象的扮演角色仍未确认。年龄，药物或潜在疾病时对准备作用的反应影响仍有待了解。再者，过多的准备作用诱发 ("hyperconditioning") 可能有害 [1,2]。

人体是可以组成各种保护、防御、适应或代偿机转，以对抗各种侵犯或压力，从而维持等稳性及正常功能。人体对很多攻击或压迫可以诱发保护，防御，适应或代偿机转，亦称「自愈功能」，从而维持体内等稳性及正常机能。造物主赋予人类两项宝贝：生命 (生理) 及防卫或代偿机转 (逆转病生理)。虽然我们不能制造生理 (生命)，但是我们可以诱发自愈功能以防卫甚而逆转疾病及老化，从而维持健康。

全身优化是生理作用，而非药物或治疗反应。所以，全身优化能恢复或逆转疾病及老化过程，以维持体内等稳性及正常机能，进而达到逆转疾病及老化。

参考文献

1. Whittaker P, Przyklenk K. From ischemic conditioning to "hyperconditioning": clinical phenomenon and basic science opportunity. Dose Response 2014 doi:10.2203/dose-response 14.03.Whittaker.
2. Johnsen J, Pryds K, Salman R et al. Optimizing the cardioprotective effects of remote ischemic preconditioning (abstr) Eur Heart J 2014;35 Suppl 1:444.

2.6 再生医学

再生医学是许多学术相关的领域，以修复，恢复或更换人体缺少，受损，异常或病变的细胞、组织或器官，使其恢复或重建正常结构及功能。它是根据与生俱来的自然自愈机能，即组织再生机能，存在于人体器官研发而来。

再生医学可分为三个主要应用方面，即细胞疗法 (Cell therapy)，组织安装 (tissue engineering) 及人造器官 (bioartificial organ)。细胞疗法是利用活细胞去修复，维持或加强组织及器官的功能。组织安装是利用细胞及支撑结构或生物分子的帮助，以重建生物组织。人造器官是用于支持主要器官如肝及肾的失能。

近期策略包括移植成体或很多效能干细胞 (adult or pluripotent stem cell) 以更换组织。有指望的研究包括刺激内源性干细胞原位修复，类器官 (organoid) 移植以修复较小的组织损伤，及利用同种类嵌合物产生的有效器官来进行移植。类器官是本体更新，本体组合，立体的细胞群包括器官特有的细胞

种类，以模拟器官功能及结构。利用同种类嵌合物产生的有效器官可以修复严重的组织缺损。宿主动物可以用来安装嵌合物以产生人类类器官适合器官移植，这一过程称为同种类嵌合体 (interspecies chimerism)。

应用再生医学可能对创伤，器官末期衰竭或其他病症病人有新的治疗。近期有疾病或创伤病人可以利用器官移植治疗，但器官捐赠者严重不足。再生医学应用干细胞、细胞移植、材料科学及医学工程以制造生物代替品，从而修复及维持疾病或创伤组织正常功能。亦即组织及器官再生以提供器官捐赠替代方案。

循环的血液细胞是经由骨髓内造血干细胞 (hematopoietic stem cell) 产生先驱血细胞 (progenitor cells) 制造。造血干细胞是多效能，具分化成所有的血液细胞如：红血球及白血球细胞、血小板、淋巴细胞等的能力。骨髓移植是治疗血癌成功的细胞治疗法第一例[1]。干细胞是有能力本体更新及分化成其他细胞。干细胞可以是全效能 (totipotent)，很多效能 (pluripotent)，多效能 (multipotent) 或单

效能 (unipotent)的。最初起源，所有干细胞源自于胚胎经过成长过程产生全效能干细胞 (胚胎及胎盘)，之后是很多效能干细胞 (胚胎)，多效能干细胞 (三层胚胎：外皮，中皮及内皮层)，单效能干细胞 (组织) 及同脉的先驱细胞 (lineage-committed progenitor cells)。干细胞可以从人体胚胎或体组织取得，或可以从己分化的体细胞诱发。干细胞具组织先驱及改善组织修复机能作用。移植的干细胞直接更替损毁组织，提供主要组件以产生新组织。以人体胚胎干细胞产生的视网膜组织移植，可以治疗视网膜退化症 (macular degeneration of retina)[2]。脐带血中的干细胞是多效能及强再生能力，应用在治疗先天性代谢疾病[3]。其他干细胞来源有羊水及胎盘。这些干细胞可以从生长中胚胎羊膜穿刺或绒毛膜抽取标本时获得，或于生产时从胎盘获得。这些干细胞可以保存作为己用或储存起来。成年干细胞丛生在身体很多组织包括骨髓，脂肪组织及血液，常常用来治疗淋巴瘤，血癌或自体免疫疾病[4]。间叶细胞 (中皮层胚胎细胞，mesenchymal cell) 可以从很多成年组织包括骨髓或脂肪组织获得，应用于非血液疾病。在缺血性，发炎性及免疫性疾病有评估间叶干细胞疗效[5]。再者，无论哪种体内细胞如从皮肤切片取得的成年纤维细胞 (在

体内形成纤维组织的结缔组织细胞，fibroblast)，亦可以诱导重整为很多效能干细胞 (induced pluripotent stem cell, iPS cell)[6]。由 iPS 干细胞产生出来的视网膜外皮细胞可以移植在老人黄斑病变 (macular degeneration)[7]。除了治疗血液疾病及烧伤外，干细胞也应用于骨科的骨移植及眼科的眼角膜移植。再者，动物实验也指出干细胞可以治疗视网膜失明，巴金森氏病，脊椎损伤，心肌梗塞及糖尿病。人体胚胎干细胞亦应用在严重心脏衰竭病人[8]。亦有胚胎干细胞临床试验在脊椎损伤，糖尿病及肌萎缩硬化症 (amyotrophic lateral sclerosis)[9]。

生物材料可以提供可携带细胞的物理输送器称为支架 (scaffold)[10]。培养上皮细胞或纤维细胞在聚合物支架上可以组成组织工程皮肤，可以移植在烧伤病人[11]。自此，以支架组合细胞成组织来进行移植变得普遍。器官和组织的脱细胞作用 (decellularization) 亦是支架来源。在组织工程中的临床应用包括皮肤，骨髓，眼角膜重建。

基因疗法 (gene therapy) 是将一种或多种外源基因 (称为转基因，transgene) 引入一种或多种细胞

类型，或操纵基因序列 (称为基因编辑，gene editing) 及操纵基因表现 (称为抑制基因表现，gene silencing)，以将好的 DNA 代替坏的 DNA。基因疗法在临床上用途有限或仍在探讨阶段，例如：遗传性疾病，先天性视网膜病变，血红素蛋白疾病，癌病等。基因疗法的主要副作用是基因毒性 (genotoxicity)，特别是发展成癌症。

血小板是众所周知的细胞因子 (炎症和免疫反应的介质，cytokine) 及生长因子 (growth factor) 来源[12,13]。自 1998 年以来，血小板衍生产品例如：富含血小板的血浆，血小板凝胶，富含血小板的纤维蛋白和血小板滴眼剂，已经在再生医学中用以改善修复组织[14,15,16]。因为他们可以重塑和收缩伤口，血小板衍生产品可以有效治疗皮肤伤口愈合，糖尿病性溃疡，不愈合的溃疡和褥疮[16,17,18]。血小板衍生物被发现可以改善骨骼成长，骨骼再生和骨密度，可以治疗肌腱和韧带断裂[19]，以及运动员的急性和慢性肌腱、韧带和肌肉损伤[20]。血小板衍生物似乎可以治疗干眼症，眼角膜溃疡(眼角膜外皮不愈合的损伤)，糖尿病性角膜炎等[21,22]。总体而言，血小板治疗的原理仍在争论中，需要更多的研究来确定其治疗功效。

目前，许多临床试验在进行中，以测试再生医学对治疗很多疾病的安全性和有效性。大多数都是利用成年干细胞进行治疗[23]。即使已经取得了显著成就，尤其是在整形外科，眼科和骨科方面，再生医学仍主要是实验阶段，到目前为止仍未达到预期效果。此外，移植干细胞有可能形成癌症。干细胞是具有自我更新 (self-renewal) 及分化 (differentiation) 能力的细胞。自我更新需进行细胞分裂 (cell division) 可能导致基因不稳定及癌变。目前，胚胎干细胞由于被移植到患者体内后很可能形成肿瘤而被排除在临床应用之外[24]。

参考文献

1. Thomas ED, Lochte HL Jr, Lu WC. Intravenous infusion of bone marrow in patients receiving radiation and chemotherapy. N Eng J Med 1957;257:491-6
2. Schwartz SD, Regillo CP, Lam BL et al. Human embryonic stem cell-derived retinal pigment epithelium in patients with age-related macular degeneration and Stargardt's macular dystrophy: follow-up of tw2o open-label phase 1/2 studies. Lancet 2015;385:509
3. Wagner JE, Gluckman E. Umbilical cord blood transplantation: the first 20 years. Semin Hematol 2010;47(1):3-12
4. Korbling M, Estrov Z. Adult stem cells for tissue repair: a new therapeutic concept? N Eng J Med 2003;349(6):570-82
5. Boregowda SV, Phinney DG. Therapeutic applications of mesenchymal stem cells: current outlook. BioDrugs 2012;26(4):201-8
6. Yamanaka S. Induced pluripotent stem cells: past, present and future. Cell stem cell 2012;10(6):678-84
7. Mandai M, Watanabe A, Kurimoto Y et al. Autologous induced stem-cell-derived retinal cells for macular degeneration,. N Eng J Med 2017;376:1038
8. Menascdhe P,Vanneaux V, Hagege Aet al. Transplantation of human embryonic stem cell derived cardiovascular progenitors for severe ischemic left ventricular dysfunction. J Am Coll Cardiol 2018;71:429
9. Trounson A, Dewitt ND. Pluripotent stem cells progressing to the clinic. Nat Rev Mol Cell Biol 2016;17:194
10. Fuchs JR, Nasseri BA, Vacanti JP. Tissue engineering: a 21st century solution to surgical reconstruction. Ann Thorac Surg 2001;72:577-91

11. Oconnor NE, Mulliken JB, Bankeschlegel S, Kehinde O, Green H. Grafting of burns with cultured epithelium prepared from autologous epidermal cells. Lancet 1981;1:75-8
12. Barrientos S, Stojadinovic O, Golinko MS et al. Growth factors and cytokines in wound healing. Wound Repair Regen 2008;15:585-601
13. Blair P, Flaumenhaft R. Platelet alpha-granules: basic biology and clinical correlates. Blood Rev 2009;23:177-89
14. Dohan Ehrenfest DM, Andia I, Zumstein MA et al. Classification of platelet concentrates 9(platelet-rich plasma-PRP, platelet-rich fibrin-PRF) for topical and infiltrative use in orthopedic and sports medicine: current consensus, clinical implications and perspectives. Muscles Ligaments Tendons J 2014;4:3-9
15. Burnouf T, Goubran HA, Chen TM et al. Blood-derived biomaterials and platelet growth factors in regenerative medicine. Blood Rev 2013;27:77-89
16. Carter MJ, Fylling CP, Parnell LK. Use of platelet rich plasma gel on wound healing: a systematic review and meta-analysis. Eplasty 2011;11:e38
17. Shan CQ, Zhang YN, Ma J et al. Evaluation of the effects of homologous platelet gel on healing lower extremity wounds in patients with diabetes. Int J Low Extrem Wounds 2013;12:22-9
18. Scerola S, Nicolette G, Brenta F et al. Allogenic platelet gel in the treatment of pressure sores: a pilot study. Int Wound J 2010;7:184-90
19. Alsouson J, Thompson M, Hulley P et al. The biology of platelet-rich plasma and its application in trauma and orthopedic surgery: a review of the literature. J Bone Joint Surg 2009;91:987-96
20. Westerlain AS, Braun HJ, Harris AH, Kim HJ, Pragor JL. The systemic effects of platelet-rich plasma injection. Am J Sports Med 2013;41:186-93

21. Kojima T, Higuchi A, Goto E et al. Autologous serum eye drops for the treatment of dry eyes disease. Cornea 2008;27:25-30
22. Jeng BH, Dupps Jr W. Autologous serum 50% eye drops in the treatment of persistent epithelial defects. Cornea 2009;28:1104-8
23. Trounson A, McDonald C. Stem cell therapies in clinical trials: progress and challenges. Cell Stem Cell 2015;17:11-22
24. Erdo F, Buhrle C, Blunk J et al. Host-dependent tumor genesis of embryonic stem cell transplantation in experimental stroke. J Cereb Blood flow Metab 2003;23:780-5

2.7 纳米医学

纳米科技包括制造及应用，如细胞内构造物及分子大小于 100 纳米的材料及装置 (以下所称之纳米粒子皆意指尺度在 100 纳米以内的材料或装置)。纳米医学 (nanomedicine) 是应用纳米科技在医学用途上。纳米医学的目的是在分子层面上，应用纳米装置及纳米材料操作及执行单一细胞的医术，从而广博的监测，控制，构造，修复，防卫及改善人体生理系统，最终达成诊断，治疗及预防疾病的医学效益。

纳米于医学方面应用很广，利用纳米微粒子 (nano particle) 为显影剂 (contrast agent) 及萤光染料 (fluorescent dye)，应用在医学影像，生物感应及化验上。纳米粒子另一主要应用是药物输送，包括脂性聚合物 (lipid-based polymers)，树枝状结晶 (dendrimers)，及病毒成分的纳米粒子 (virus-based nanoparticles)。纳米粒子及纳米输送系统可以改善药物吸收，药物指定作用在疾病组织所在处，及允许药物释放预定时间。这些装置是可以减少药物剂量，增加药物到达目标组织程度 (bioavailability) 及减少药物副作用。

纳米粒子的大小及形状有不一样的物理化学、生物、电磁、磁场、光效应、热能及能量性质及效能，所以提供很多保健效益[1]。在中或大量时，纳米粒子可引起较强药理作用；在小剂量时，纳米粒子能提升非药理性能、生理性代偿机转、及体内防卫机转[2-5]。作为轻微的外界刺激，植物、矿物质或动物来源的天然、非药物纳米粒子可以调整及加强生理代偿机转，加强神经及免疫系统机能。

因为其加强的化学活性，纳米粒子可与空气及水中污染物反应，转变成无害物质。例如含小量钯 (Palladium) 的纳米粒子可以改变地下水源的有害物质转换成无害物质。

超过 200 年的顺势医学 (homeopathy medicine)，可能是一种古老及安全的纳米疗法。顺势医学药物的制造方法 (磨碎、重复演替、玻璃器具、稀释、手工移动稀释步骤)，可能导致各种纳米粒子体积及形状，所以有不同特性。近期研究指出因为其制造方法过程，顺势医学药物可能含有二氧化矽 (silica) 及/或其他物质的纳米粒子。顺势医学是利用低剂量矿物质、植物及/或动物来源的纳米粒子能量达到治疗各

种疾病[6,7]。

应用纳米科技于日常生活的产品有超过上千种如：衣服、床具，体育用品，鞋，化妆品及杀菌剂等等。

纳米科技的原理是正常体积的物质在纳米尺度下会有不同及有效的性质及效能。经由制造出非常细小的纳米粒子，可以增加体表面积与其他物质相互作用，从而增加反应及吸附能力，具有独特的电磁，化学，生物及能量性质，提供很多健康益处。

纳米粒子覆盖物产生纳米结构表面，可以经由物理作用刺破附着的细菌细胞，从而有效杀菌[8]。纳米粒子本身亦具有强大杀菌功能，主要经由三种机转如：氧化刺激 (oxidative stress)，非氧化刺激 (non-oxidative stress) 及金属离子释出 (metal ion release)[9]。当应用于缝合线及绷带材质时候，抗菌的纳米包敷料可以预防或治疗感染。利用纳米包敷料及缝合线，近期纳米科技于医学上应用以加强烧伤病人伤口愈合。

纳米粒子包敷料或纺织品是自我清洁，光能动力或鲜艳色彩，防退色，防皱，防磨损，防污，杀菌消毒，减少异味，过滤污染物及抗辐射等特性。

因为其纳米体积，纳米粒子可以和生物系统相互作用。当纳米粒子内在化 (internalize) 在细胞时，它们会被察觉为有毒的或外来的异物，所以可能分别地诱发自噬及免疫机能[10]。自噬机能经由分解各种过多或无用的细胞内蛋白质及小器官物质，可以加强排毒机能，从而维持细胞等稳性 (cellular homeostasis)[10]。自噬机能也在免疫及分解细胞内病原菌扮演一重要角色[11]。所以纳米科技可以优化及加强细胞排毒及免疫机能。

刺激物 (stress) 是所有能影响等稳性的物理，化学，电磁，感染，心理与社会或生物因素。纳米粒子是对生物显著，奇特及外来异物的轻微细胞刺激物，可以诱发适应及代偿机转，从而优化及保护身体以维持细胞等稳性及身体机能[12,13]。

到目前为止，纳米医学对很多疾病包括老化，心血管及癌病变诊断，治疗及预防具有革命性的前景。

参考文献

1. Roduner E. Size matters: why nanomaterials are different. Chem Soc Rev 2006;35(7):583-92
2. Bell IR, Koithan M, Brooks AJ. Testing nanoparticle-allostatic cross-adaptation-sensitization mode for homeopathic remedy effects. Homeopathy 2013,in press
3. Bell IR, Howerter A, Jackson N, Brooks AJ, Schwartz GE. Multi-week resting EEG cordance change patterns from repeated olfactory activation with two constitutionally-salient homeopathic remedies in healthy young adults. J Alternative Complementary Medicine 2012;18:445-53
4. Bell IR, Koithan M. A model for homeopathic remedy effects: low dose nanoparticles, allostatic cross-adaptation, and time-dependent sensitization in a complex adaptive system. BMC Complementary Alternative Medicine 2012;12(1):191
5. Bell IR, Schwartz GE. Adaptive network nanomedicine: an integrated model for homeopathic medicine. Frontiers Bioscience 2013;5(2):685-708
6. Chikramare PS, Suresh AK, Bellare JR, Kane SG. Extreme homeopathic dilutions retain starting materials: a nanoparticulate perspective. Homeopathy 2010;99:231-42
7. Upadhyay RP, Nayak C. Homeopathy emerging as nanomedicine. Int J High Dilution Res 2011;10:299-310
8. Yuan Y, Zhang Y. Enhanced biomimic bactericidal surfaces by coating with positively-charged ZIF nano-dagger arrays. Nanomedicine 2017;13:2199-2207
9. Zaidi S, Misba L, Khan AV. Nanoparticles: a revolution in infection control in post antibiotic era. Nanomedicine 2017;13:2281-2301
10. Boyle KB, Randow F. The role of eat-me signals and autophagy cargo receptors in innate immunity. Curr Opin Microbiol 2013;16:339-48.
11. Popp L, Segatori L. Differential autophagic response to nano-sized materials. Current Opinion Biotechnology 2015;36:129-36.
12. Bell IR, Koithan M. A model for homeopathic remedy effects: low dose nanoparticles, allostatic cross-adaptation, and time-dependent sensitization in a complex adaptive system. BMC Complem Altern Med 2012;12(1):191

13. Bell IR, Schwartz GE. Adaptive network nanomedicine: an integrated model for homeopathic medicine. Front Biosci 2013;5(2):685-708

2.8 氧气疗法

高压氧疗法

高压氧气是在 100%氧气的环境中，施加大于一个大气压力。这导致氧气分压增加，与基于两种气体定律 (Boyle 和 Henry 定律) 的压力增加成比例。这样氧气分压及组织的氧气供应增加。高压氧可增加血中氧浓度，以满足组织氧气需求。当患者在高压舱中时，氧气通过肺部输送至全身。

高压氧疗法可作为多种医学状况的主要或辅助疗法[1,2]，包括一氧化碳或氰化物中毒[2]，潜水夫病 (减压损伤) 及空气栓塞[2]，严重贫血，急性创伤或烧伤 如压碎创伤，腔隙创伤症候群 (compartment syndrome)，血管损伤[3]，放射损伤[4]，感染[5]，气性坏疽 (gas gangrene)，颅内脓肿，坏死性软组织感染，难治性骨髓炎，难愈性溃疡，皮肤移植和伤口愈合[3]，感觉神经性失聪等[6]。其他高压氧疗法包括冠心病，系统发炎反应症候群 (systemic inflammatory syndrome)，脑部或脊髓损伤，镰状细胞性贫血 (sickle cell disease)，冻伤，肌风湿病

(fibromyalgia)，脑中风等都有功效 [1,7-10]。

高压氧疗法的禁忌症包括未经治疗的气胸，阻塞性肺疾病，上呼吸道或鼻窦感染，近期耳部或胸部手术，未治疗的发烧等 [11]。高压氧疗法通常是安全的及耐受性良好。高压氧疗法的副作用包括中耳气压损伤，鼻窦气压损伤，可逆性近视，肺气压损伤，肺氧气中毒，癫痫发作等 [12]。

高压氧具有抗发炎和抗氧化作用，可减少自由基的产生及增加一氧化氮的产生 [13]。这些作用是由于减少白血球增加及活化，水肿，细胞坏死，及增强抗氧化酶的功效 [14]。高压氧可改善组织氧和吞噬作用 (phagocytosis, 清除在感染、炎症或伤口修复过程中积累的微生物或组织废弃物)，损坏细菌代谢，抑制外毒素的产生及增强抗生素效应 [15]。高压氧诱发自由基 (reactive oxygen species) 产生及过度氧化压力 (oxidative stress) 从而损伤肿瘤。

与缺血性前准备作用类似，高压氧会引起轻度的氧化压力，从而诱发缺血性耐受性，并通过抗氧化作用，和氧作用 (hyperoxygenation)，血管收缩 [16] 及

自噬机能 [17]，以保护缺血/再灌流引起的损伤。 高压氧前及后准备作用可以减少心脏，脑，肝及肾脏的缺血/再灌流损伤 [18-21]。

超氧疗法

臭氧 (ozone) 与氧气一样，是最强氧化剂之一。 像其他气体一样，臭氧必须溶解于水中，才能与有机物质相互作用。 臭氧溶解于水之后，能快速地分解成一系列超氧活性氧自由基 (reactive oxygen species) 包括二氧化氢 (hydrogen peroxide)，超氧化阴离子 (superoxide anion)，氧化自由基 (hydroxyl radical) 及低氯酸 (Hypochlorous acid) [22,23]。

超氧的氧化化学过程会产生二氧化氢。 该二氧化氢进入细胞从而产生各种作用。 在红血球中，超氧会增强血液中的血红素释放氧气 [24]。 在白血球及血管内皮细胞中，超氧可以刺激白介素 (interleukins，炎症和免疫反应的介质，例如肿瘤坏死因子，白介素 IL-1)，干扰素 (interferons，对病毒感染有抵抗力的蛋白质)，生长因子及一氧化氮 (nitric oxide) 的产生 [25,26]。

在血小板中，超氧有利于生长因子的释放[27,28]。在其他细胞类型如巨噬细胞(macrophages)，呼吸道上皮细胞中，超氧可刺激活化细胞，细胞因子(cytokines)分泌及经由其氧化作用(pro-oxidant action)，诱发长期的抗氧化系统效能[29,30]。

缺血性前准备作用是一种可诱导的有效体内机制。通过这机制，短暂的缺血/再灌流可以优化及保护之后持续的缺血/再灌流损伤。另一方面，已证实低剂量超氧，可以诱发中等程度的氧化压力，从而诱发缺血性耐受性及优化体内抗氧化系统[31]。这机制也可优化及保护之后持续的缺血/再灌流损伤。超氧可导致对慢性氧化压力的有效适应性[32]。超氧可经由适应氧化压力，从而促进氧化前准备作用(oxidative preconditioning)，以防止因自由基引起的损伤[32,33,34]。

超氧前及后准备作用能保护心脏，肺，肝，肾，肠，肌肉等各种器官和组织缺血/再灌流损伤[35-38]。超氧也能提升一氧化氮的产生，减少组织氧化压力指标(如脂质过氧化 lipid peroxidation，蛋白质氧化 protein oxidation 及亚硝酸盐和硝酸盐 nitrite plus nitrate)，及增强抗氧化酶的活性[39]。超氧可以调整抗氧化酶，一氧化氮机转[40]及其他细胞作用机转从而对很多疾病有治疗效果。因具有抗氧化和抗发炎特性，超氧可改善血液循环和缺氧组织的氧气供应，增强免疫功能和释出生长因子，通过改善氧气供给来增强一般新陈代谢，并可以诱导生理功能机转[41,42]。超氧疗法的治疗应用有激活免疫系统以治疗感染病[43]、老化及癌病[44,45]、慢性退化性疾病包括神经退化性疾病[46]、慢性肝病和类风湿性关节炎、减少血管疾病的发炎及缺氧[27,40,47]、下背痛[48]、激活神经内分泌系统以诱发神经系统保护作用，从而获得健康及生活品质的改善。

超氧在各种皮肤疾病[49]、烧伤和伤口愈合[50]具有局部治疗效果。因具有杀菌特性而被应用在对食物及水进行杀菌消毒[51]。超氧对细菌、霉菌及病毒[52]具有很强的抗菌作用，并可能增强抗生素的杀菌及抑菌作用。

应用一种可以诱发糖尿病的抗生素streptozotocin，以测试超氧对糖尿病的保护效果进行研究。发现超氧疗法可以改善血糖控制，可分解

糖，保护胰脏及防止氧化损伤[53]。此外，超氧的抗氧化特性保护胰脏 beta 细胞功能及降低高血糖[54]。这些研究结果指出超氧可帮助治疗糖尿病及其并发症。

超氧可增强对缺氧组织的氧气、糖及能量 ATP 的供给，并导致血管扩张，增加一氧化氮，刺激血管增生并提供免疫调节作用[55]。可诱导不同细胞类型中抗氧化酶的上调，从而有效地重新平衡「氧化 - 抗氧化」的不平衡[56]。

超氧可抑制肺、乳腺和子宫肿瘤细胞的生长，因此在癌症中可能具有治疗效果[46]。另外超氧对结肠癌细胞有直接毒性杀伤作用[57]。

参考文献

1. Gill AL, Bell CN. Hyperbaric oxygen: its use, mechanisms of action and outcome. QJM 2004;97:385
2. Leach RM,l Rees PJ, Wilmshurst P. Hyperbaric oxygen therapy. BMJ 1998;317:1140
3. Wattel F, Mathieu D, Neviere R, Bocquillon N. Acute peripheral ischemia and compartment syndromes: a role for hyperbaric oxygenation. Anesthesia 1998;53 suppl 2:63
4. Mustoe TA, Porres-Reyes BH. Modulation of wound healing response in chronic irradiated tissues. Clin Plast Surg 1993;20:465
5. Kaye D. Effect of hyperbaric oxygen on Clostridia in vitro and in vivo. Proc Soc Exp Biol Med 1967;124:360
6. Chin CS, Lee TY, Wu MF. Adjunctive hyperbaric oxygen treatment for idiopathic sudden sensorineural hearing loss. Undersea Hyperb Med 2017;44:63
7. Sharifi M, Fares W, Abdel-Karim I et al. Usefulness of hyperbaric oxygen therapy to inhibit restenosis after percutaneous coronary intervention for acute myocardial infarction or unstable angina pectoris. Am J Cardil 2004;93:1533
8. Rusyniak DE, Kirk MA, May JD et al. Hyperbaric oxygen therapy in acute ischemic stroke: results of the hyperbaric oxygen in acute ischemic stroke trial pilot study. Stroke 2003;34:571
9. Yildiz S, Kiralp MZ, Akin A et al. A new treatment for fibromyalgia syndrome: hyperbaric oxygen therapy. J Int Med Res 2004;32:263
10. Higdon B, Youngman L, Regehr M, Chiou S. Deep frostbite treated with hyperbaric oxygen and thrombolytic therapies. Wounds 2015;27:215
11. Toklu AS, Korpinar S, Erelel M et al. Are pulmonary bleb and bullae a contraindication for hyperbaric oxygen treatment? Respir Med 2008;102:1145

12. Camporesi EM, Bosco G. Mechanisms of action of hyperbaric oxygen therapy. Undersea Hyperb Med 2014;41:247
13. Thackham JA, McElwain DL, Long RJ. The use of hyperbaric oxygen therapy to treat chronic wounds: a review. Wound Repair Regen 2008;16:321
14. MacFarlance C, Crouje FC. Hyperbaric oxygen and surgery. S Afr J Surg 2001;39:117
15. Dauwe PB, Pulikkottil BJ, Lavery L et al. Does hyperbaric oxygen therapy work in facilitating acute wound healing: a systematic review. Plast Reconstr Surg 2014;133:208e-15e
16. Nylander G, Lewis DH, Nordstrom H et al. Reduction of postischemic edema with hyperbaric oxygen. Plast Reconstr Surg 1985;76:596
17. Yan W, Zhang H, Bai X, Lu Y, Dong H, Xiong L. Autophagy activation is involved in neuroprotection induced by hyperbaric oxygen preconditioning against focal cerebral ischemia in rats. Brain Res 2011;1402:109-121
18. Stavitsky Y, Shandling AH, Ellestad MH et al. Hyperbaric oxygen and thrombolysis in myocardial infarction: The "HOT MI" randomized multicenter study. Cardiology 1998;90:131
19. Xiong L, Zhu Z, Dong H et al. Hyperbaric oxygen preconditioning induces neuroprotection against ischemia in transient not permanent middle cerebral artery occlusion rat model. Chin Med J 2000;113(9):836-9
20. Gurer A, Ozdagean M, Gomceli I et al. Hyperbaric oxygenation attenuates renal ischemia-reperfusion injury in rats. Transplant Proc 2006;38:3337
21. Ramalho RJ, de Oliveira PST, Caraglieri RC et al. Hyperbaric oxygen therapy induces kidney protection in an ischemia/reperfusion model in rats. Transplant Proc 2012;44:2333-6

22. Bocci V. Ozone therapy may act as a biological response modifier in cancer. Forch Komplement 1998;5:54-60
23. Bocci V, Valacchi G, Corradeschi F et al. Studies on the biological effects of ozone: Generation of reactive oxygen species (ROS) after exposure of human blood to ozone. J Biol Regulat Homeost Agent 1998;12:67-75
24. Freeman BA, Mudd JB. Reaction of ozone with sulphydryls of human erythrocyte. Arch Biochem Biophys 1981;208:212-20
25. Bocci V, Luzzi E, Corradeshi F et al. Studies on the biological effects of ozone: Cytokine production and glutathione levels in human erythrocytes. J Biol Regulat Homeost Agent 1998;12:67-75
26. De Groote D. Direct stimulation of cytokine (IL-1B, TNF, IL6, *IL2, IFNg and* GM-CFS) in whole blood. Cytokine 1992;4:239-48
27. Bocci V, Valacchi G, Rossi D et al. Studies on the biological effects of ozone: effects of ozone on human platelets. Platelets 1999;10:110-6
28. Bocci V, Valacchi G, Corradeschi F, Fanetti G. Studies on the biological effects of ozone: effects on the total antioxidant status and on interleukin 8 production. Mediat Inflam 1998;7:313-7
29. Hamilton RF, Hazbun ME, Jumper CA. 4-hydroxynonenal mimics ozone-induced modulation of macrophages function ex vivo. Am J Respir Cell Mol Biol 1996;15:275-82
30. Jaspers I, Flescher E, Chen LC. Ozone-induced IL8 expression and transcription factor binding in respiratory epithelial cells. Am J Physiol 1997;272:504-511
31. Clavien PA, Yadar S, Sindram D, Bentley RC. Protective effects of ischemic preconditioning for liver resection performed under inflow occlusion in humans. Ann Surg 2000;232:155-62
32. Leon OS, Menendez S, Merino N et al. Ozone oxidative preconditioning: a protection against cellular damage by free radicals. Mediat Inflam 1998;7:289-94
33. Peralta C, Leon OS, Xaus C et al. Protective effect of ozone treatment on the injury associated with hepatic ischemia-reperfusion: antioxidant-prooxidant balance. Free Radical Res

1999;31:191-6
34. Barber E, Menendez S, Leon OS et al. Prevention of renal injury after induction of ozone tolerance in rats submitted to warm ischemia. Mediators Inflam 1999;8:37-41
35. Ozkan H, Ekinci S, Uysal B et al. Evaluation and comparison of the effect of hypothermia and ozone on ischemia-reperfusion injury of skeletal muscle in rats. J Surg Res 2015;196:313-9
36. Deljado-Roche L, Martinez-Sanchez G, Re L. Ozone oxidative preconditioning prevents atherosclerosis development in New Zealand White rabbits. Cardiovas Pharmacol 2013;61:160-5
37. Isik A, Peker K, Gursul C et al. The effect of ozone and naringin on intestinal ischemia/reperfusion injury in an experimental model. Int J Surg 2015;21:38-44
38. Gao C, Sun X, Zhang G et al. Hyperoxygenated solution preconditioning attenuates lung injury induced by intestinal ischemia reperfusion in rabbits. J Surg Res 2008;146:24-31
39. Ajaurieh HH, Berlanga J, Merino N et al. Role of protein oxidation in the protection conferred by ozone-oxidative-preconditioning in hepatic ischemia/reperfusion. Transpl Int 2005;18:604-12
40. Valacchi G, Bocci V. Studies on the biological effects of ozone: release of factors from human endothelial cells. Mediators Inflam 2000;9:271-6
41. Bocci V. Is it true that ozone is always toxic? The end of a dogma. Toxicol Appl Pharmacol 2006;216(3):493-504
42. Sagai M, Bocci V. Mechanisms of action involved in ozone therapy: is healing induced via a mild oxidative stress? Med Gas Res 2011;1:29
43. Hatch GE. Commentary on cellular, biochemical and functional effects of ozone: new research and perspectives on ozone health effects. Toxicol Lett 1990;51:119-20
44. Sanhueza PA, Reed GD, Davis WT, Miller TL. An environmental decision-making tool for evaluating ground-level ozone-related health effects. J Air Waste Manage Assoc 2003;53:1448-59
45. Sweet F, Kao MS, Lee S. Ozone selectively inhibits growth of human cancer cells. Science 1980;209:931-3

46. Re L, Mawsouf MN, Menendez S et al. Ozone therapy: clinical and basic evidence of its therapeutic potential. Arch Med Res 2008;39:17-26
47. Los M, Droge W, Striker K et al. Hydrogen peroxide as a potent activator of T-lymphocyte functions. Eur J Immunol 1995;25:159-65
48. Andreula CF, Simonetti L, De Santis F et al. Minimally invasive oxygen-ozone therapy for lumbar disc herniation. Am J Neuroradiol 2003;24:996-1000
49. Aubourg P. L'ozone medicale: production, posologie, models d'applications cliniques. Bull Med Paris 1938;52:745-9
50. Valacchi G, Lim Y, Belmonte G et al. Ozonated sesame oil enhances cutaneous wound healing in SKH1 mice. Wound Repair Regener 2010;19:107-115
51. Moore G, Griffith C, Peters A. Bactericidal properties of ozone and its potential application as a terminal disinfectant. J Food Prot 2000;63:1100-6
52. Kim JG, Yousef AE, Dave S. Application of ozone for enhancing the microbiological safety and quality of foods: a review. J Food Prot 1999;62:1071-87
53. Al-Dalain SM,l Martinez-Sanchez G, Candelano-Jalil E et al. Ozone treatment reduces biomarkers of oxidative and endothelial damage in an experimental diabetes model in rats. Pharmacol Res 2001;44:391-6
54. Martinez-Sanchez G, Al-Dalain SM, Menendez S et al. Ozone treatment reduces blood oxidative stress and pancreas damaged in a streptocotocin-induced diabetes model in rats. Acta Farm Boraerence 2005;24:491-7
55. Tasdoven GE, Derin AT, Yaprak N, Ozeaglar HV. The place of hyperbaric oxygen therapy and ozone therapy in sudden hearing loss. Braz J Otorhinolaryngol 2017;83(4):457-63
56. Di Paolo N, Gaggiotti E, Galli F. Extracorporeal blood oxygenation and ozonation: clinical and biological implications of ozone therapy. Redox Rep 2005;10:121-30
57. Simonetti V, Quagliariello V, Giustetto P et al. Association of ozone with 5-fluorouracil and cisplatin in regulation of human

colon cancer cell viability: in vitro anti-inflammatory properties of ozone in colon cancer cells exposed to lipopolysaccharides. Evidence-based Complementary Alternative Med 2017;2017:7414083

2.9 益生菌 益菌生 益生菌合并剂

人体肠道栖居着佰万兆的微生物，称为肠道微生态(gut microbiota)及其基因称为肠道微生基因(gut microtome)与宿主共栖共生。这肠道微生态包括几佰微生物种，佰万基因及很多新陈代谢机能。肠道微生态对宿主的等稳性(homeostasis)，生理及健康是有益的。微生态有定植、定量的特性，除了栖居于肠道外，亦会栖居于身体其他器官如：呼吸道，皮肤，口腔及尿道等。微生态会因为个人的饮食，生活方式，感染，免疫反应等因素而随时改变。

已清楚知道肠道微生态对宿主生理有很多影响，诸如对宿主的免疫控制，营养，生长及肠道等稳性有重要作用。很多急性或慢性疾病与栖居的微生态定值种类的改变有关，称为肠道微生态失衡(intestinal dysbiosis)[1]。在生理情况下，肠道微生态能激活免疫系统，特别是经过肠道相关的淋巴组织。再者，肠道微生态也能激活T及B淋巴细胞及免疫球蛋白。肠道微生态能减少因表皮损伤如抗生素、高脂饮食、化疗、高血压等引起的肠道渗透性增加。肠道微生态能改变新陈代谢包括处理不被消化纤维，产生

短链脂肪酸 (short-chain fatty acids)，维生素，矿物质，胆汁酸 (bile acids) 及降低血脂肪。肠道微生态能诱发自噬机转 (autophagy，细胞清除细胞废弃物的机转以维持细胞等穩性) 及产生抗微生物胜肽、蛋白质及脂肪蛋白以限制病菌衍生；能改变骨质细胞机能及质量，以维持骨骼等稳性及健康[2]。肠道微生态能直接产生神经内分泌代谢产物 (类荷尔蒙代谢产物如：短链脂肪酸、神经介质 neurotransmitter、肠道荷尔蒙)，神经活化引导物质如：tryptophan、kynurenine 及间接调控发炎反应，免疫反应及释出荷尔蒙，以影响神经内分泌机能[3]。

与年老相关的肠道微生态失衡证实是导致很多年老相关疾病如：慢性发炎[4]，神经退化[5]，认知障碍[6]，虚弱[7]，糖尿病[8]，肝及心血管疾病[9]及癌症[10]的重要原因。调整肠道微生态能减少发炎反应及改善免疫反应，从而减少免疫衰退(immunosenescence)。

活性益生菌 (probiotic) 食品配方是对宿主健康有益的如：乳酸杆菌 (lactobacilli) 及双歧杆菌 (bifidobacteria)。益生菌是以营养补充或食品供应。益生菌维持肠道微生态平衡及稳定，以改善消化机能

如：控制肠道输送时间，营养可用率及调整消化系统功能。研究指出益生菌对癌症，抗生素引起的腹泻，旅行常见的腹泻过敏，乳糖不耐症 (lactose intolerance)，高血压，免疫机能及维生素合成有正向效果[11]。益生菌改善肠道防御机能，调整免疫系统及产生神经介质，改善肠道微生态，消化及神经通讯系统 (gut-brain axis) 机能[12]。亦可以降低胆固醇，发炎介体 (inflammatory mediators)，血糖，血压及体重指数 (body mass index、BMI)[13]。虽然益生菌的功效在动物试验中证实，但在人体试验结果却不理想。大部分只是临床初期或小规模试验，其分子机转仍不清楚。

益菌生 (prebiotic) 是不被消化的食品配方如：非淀粉多糖体及寡糖，可以引起宿主肠道有益益生态的生长或机能而改善健康。益生菌合并剂 (symbiotic) 是益生菌和益菌生的组合配方。

益生菌是十分安全的。轻微的副作用包括口干，便秘，腹胀，呕吐，腹痛，皮肤疹及腹泻。严重的副作用在虚弱病人中少见。包括在心血管手术病人引起的败血症，过敏的病人引起严重过敏反应。年老

免疫力差的病人引起霉菌血症，及对感染产生抗生素抗药性等 [14,15]。

健康人服用益生菌，益菌生，或益生菌合并剂有否益处? Khaless 等详查医学文献结论指出，它们只有次要及短期效益。目前仍未有具体证实服用它们有何好处或效益。虽然基础研究或许有宣称它们有效，但是临床试验却不支持，而也没有证据指出服用它们能改善健康。很少人体试验指出它们有益，而目前医界并无推荐其处方使用。此外，仅肠道微生态变化并不能自动保证有益健康。虽然健康或年老人持续服用益生菌，益菌生或益生菌合并剂或许对健康有点益处，但其补充可能与补充综合维生素建议一样。亦即是说，它们对特定的对象或情况可能有益 [16]。

参考文献

1. Kim D, Zeng MY, Nunez G. The interplay between host immune cells and gut microbiota in chronic inflammatory disease. Exp Mol Med 2017;49(5):9339
2. Vaiserman AM. Gut microbiota: A player in aging and a target for anti-aging intervention. Ageing Res Review 2017;35:36-45
3. Cussotto S, Sandhu KV, Dinan TG, Cryan JF. The neuroendocrinology of the microbiota-gut-brain axis: a behavioral perspective. Frontiers Neuroendocrinol 2018;51:80-101
4. Rehman T. Role of the gut microbiota in age-related chronic inflammation. Endocr Metab Immune Disord Drug Targets 2012;12(4):361-7
5. Friedland RP. Mechanisms of molecular mimicry involving the microbiota in neurodegeneration. J Alzheimers Ds 2015;45(2):349-62
6. Magnusson KR, Havck L, Jeffrey BM et al. Relationships between diet-related changes in gut microbiome and cognitive flexibility. Neurosci 2015;300:128-40
7. Meehan CJ, Langille MG, Beiko RG. Frailty and the microbiome. Interdiscp Top Gerontol Geriatr 2015;41:54-65
8. Paun A, Danska JS. Modulation of type 1 and type 2 diabetes risk by the intestinal microbiome. Pediatr Diabetes 2016;17(7):469-77
9. Sanduzzin Zamparelli M, Compare D, Coccoli P et al. The metabolic role of gut microbiota in the development of nonalcoholic fatty liver disease and cardiovascular disease. Int J Mol Sci 2016;17(8):pii:E1225
10. Pope JL, Tomkouch S, Yang Y, Jobin C. Microbiota as a mediator of cancer progression and therapy. Transl Res

2017;179:139-54
11. Rostami FM, Mousari H, Mousari MRN et al. Efficacy of probiotics in prevention and treatment of infectious disease. Clin Microbiology Newsletter 2018;40(12):97-103
12. Sanchez B, Delgado S, Blanco-Miguez A, Lourenco A, Gueimonde M, Margolles A. Probiotics, gut microbiota and their influence on host health and disease. Mol Nutr Food Res 2017;61:1-15
13. Thushara RM, Gangadaran S, Solati Z, Moghadasian MH. Cardiovascular benefits of probiotics: a review of experimental and clinical studies. Food Funct 2016;7(2):632-42
14. Doron S, Snydman DR. Risk and safety of probiotics. Clin Infect Ds 2015;60(suppl 2):S129-234
15. Venugopalan V, Shriner KA, Wong-Beringer A. Regulatory oversight and safety of probiotic use. Infect Dis 2010;16:1661-5
16. Khalesi S, Bellissimo N, Vandelanotte C et al. A review of probiotic supplementation in healthy adults: helpful or hype? Eur J Clin Nutr 2019;73:24-37

2.10 植物营养素

植物性食物中的成分除了基础的碳水化合物、蛋白质、脂肪、维生素、矿物质、膳食纤维等营养素之外，还含有很多天然有机活性化学成分，这些植物化学物质总称为「植物营养素」（phytonutrients）。

植物营养素并不直接参与植物或真菌的生长、发育、或繁殖，因此被归类为植物衍生的代谢产物。这些化学物质是有助于保护植物免受细菌，真菌，虫子和其他威胁的侵害。

不同的植物含有不同的植物营养素(植物化学物质, phytochemicals)，这也是让植物呈现不同的色彩、气味和风味原因。

尽管这些天然生物活性化合物的植物营养素不被认为具有营养价值，它们与植物性食物中所含的维生素和矿物质不同，对人类生命体而言，他们并不是维持生命的必需品，但是这些食物在烹饪过程中以及身体在消化这些食物时，这些植物营养素会转变成其他化学物质，而参与身体的正常运转，它们可以激活

防御性细胞反应，例如自噬机能 (细胞清除细胞废弃物的机转以维持细胞等穩性)、DNA 修复及激活抗氧化酶，从而改善健康和延长寿命[1]。

几乎所有的植物性的食物及植物性制品中都含有其独特的植物营养素，包括：各种不同颜色的蔬菜水果类、全谷类、坚果 (种子) 类、豆类、茶类、根茎类食物及其他以植物为原料的植物性制品等。

植物营养素已经被证实具有抗氧化，抗发炎，抗菌，抗血脂，降血压，降血糖，抗癌，免疫调节，抗过敏，镇痛，保肝，保护皮肤及神经系统等特性[2,3]。

植物营养素通过抑制肠道有害菌，及增加有益菌如乳酸杆菌与双歧杆菌的生长，来调整肠道微生态，从而改善肠道健康[4,5]。

被发现于植物中的植物营养素有很多种类，常见的例如 :

◎ 类胡萝卜素 (carotenoids)：是抗氧化剂，可防止某些癌症，心脏病及眼部黄斑病变。

它们包括常见的如：

* α-胡萝卜素能促进视力，免疫功能，皮肤及骨骼健康

* β-胡萝卜素具有抗衰老作用，可降低癌症风险，改善肺功能，并减少糖尿并发症；

* 叶黄素 (lutein) 能降低白内障，黄斑病变及癌症的风险；

* 番茄红素可降低前列腺癌和心脏病的风险；

* 玉米黄质可防止黄斑病变，以及预防肾癌、卵巢癌和乳腺癌的风险。

一般黄色、橙色和红颜色的水果和蔬菜是类胡萝卜素含量较多的食物来源如：红番茄、西瓜、南瓜、甜红椒、胡萝卜、粉葡萄柚、柑橘类水果、地瓜、辣椒、茄子、柿子、植物香料、甜菜根、棕榈油、哈密瓜、芒果…等。

◎ 黄酮类化合物 (flavonoids)：又称类黄酮，是植物次生代谢产物的大家族，广泛存在于自然界的

植物中，具有很多药用价值的化合物，有提高动物机体抗氧化及清除自由基的能力，绝大多数植物体内都含有黄酮类化合物。

类黄酮化合物，存在于许多水果和花朵中的植物色素，生物类黄酮是植物中发现的多酚化合物质。富含于苹果、浆果、羽衣甘蓝、洋葱等、可可亚、绿茶、葡萄酒、种子或是植物根。

* 大豆和其他豆科植物中被发现含有很多异黄酮。大豆异黄酮素的结构和女性动情激素类似，可作为雌激素，缓解更年期并发症，并降低患心脏病的风险、动脉硬化、前列腺癌和雌激素相关疾病的风险；

◎吲哚 (indole) - 预防癌症。

◎木脂素 (lignans) - 可预防糖尿病，癌症和心脏病等疾病。

◎皂苷 (saponins) - 豆类（大豆，豆类，豌豆，小扁豆，羽扇豆等）是主要的皂苷类食物。可以抗发炎、降低血浆胆固醇水平。因此，它们在人类饮食中可能对降低冠心病风险很重要。

◎有机硫化学物 (organosulfur compounds) - 可刺激免疫细胞并降低癌症风险。有机硫化合物富含于洋葱、大蒜、韭菜、青花菜、番茄、酵母等。

◎ 多酚 (polyphenols) - 可预防心血管疾病和癌症。咖啡可能是人类饮食中多酚最高的来源[1]，咖啡中的多酚可激活肝脏，肌肉和心脏中的自噬机能[7]。姜黄素是印度咖哩中的一种多酚，可通过诱发自噬机能改善心脏功能[8]。

多酚具有很强的抗氧化作用，常见的多酚化合物有：儿茶素、绿原酸、异黄酮、花青素、可可多酚、姜黄素、柠檬黄素绿茶、葡萄及深色的蔬果都是多酚类物质的一个来源。

◎白藜芦醇（resveratrol）：抗氧化的多酚化合物，富含于花生、大豆、红葡萄酒、蓝莓皮、树莓皮、桑葚皮、葡萄皮等蔬果。白藜芦醇可激活自噬机能并降低老年痴呆的风险。它还具抗发炎、抗氧化、抗癌、抗老化、抗病毒、抗血小板凝集、保护心血管和神经系统的特性。它还可以降低血糖，改善肝功能

，减少过敏和哮喘病引发的炎症，保护肺部免受污染物污染，并预防癌症[8]。

◎单萜(monoterpenes)、萜烯（Terpenes）- 可降低乳腺癌和结肠癌的风险[2]。

许多植物营养素在生理功能上会产生双相的反应，即在低剂量时，具有益作用，而在高剂量时候产生有害作用。因此植物营养素的剂量决定了这些化合物产生有益还是有害作用[1]。主要必需的营养如胺基酸、维生素及矿物质也分别在低剂量和高剂量下产生双相反应[1]。所以，需要进行进一步的研究，以确定食物中或作为饮食补充剂的植物营养素的最佳剂量和使用频率。

由于缺乏明确具体性及需要较长的治疗时间，植物营养素并未列入为医药。饮食中植物营养素的最佳剂量，添加形式或方法尚未确定，近期研究并不支持补充植物营养素的益处。在未有临床验证植物营养素的益处之前，可能只鼓励人们食用含有充裕植物营养素的饮食。

参考文献

1. Martel J, Ojcins DM, Ko YF et al. Hormetic effects of phytochemicals on health and longevity. Trends Endocrin Meta 2019;30(6):335-46
2. Mann N. Phytochemicals: the colors of the new millennium. Access 2010;24:42
3. Patel S. Phytochemicals for taming agitated immune-endocrine-neural axis. Biomedicine Pharmacotherapy 2017;91:767-775
4. Kawabata K, Yoshioka Y, Terao J. Role of intestinal microbiota in the bioavailability and physiological functions of dietary polyhenols. Molecules 2019;24:e370
5. Pei R, Liu X, Bolling B. Flavonoids and gut health. Current Opinion Biotechnology 2020;61:153-9
6. Vingtdeux V et. al. AMP-activated protein kinase signaling activation by resveratrol modulates amyloid-beta peptide metabolism. J Biol Chem 2010;285:9100-13
7. Pietrocoia F et al. Coffee induces autophagy in vivo. Cell cycle 2014;13:1987-94
8. Yao Q et al. Curcumin protects against diabetic cardiomyopathy by promoting autophagy and alleviating apoptosis. J Mol Cell Cardiol 2018;124:26-34

2.11 荷尔蒙替代疗法

科学文献建议，补充雌激素，孕激素，睾丸激素，生长激素和甲状腺激素的荷尔蒙可能会改善生活品质，并预防或逆转与衰老相关的症状，包括疲劳，抑郁，体重增加，虚弱，骨质疏松和心脏病。

对于女性而言，与年龄相关的重大荷尔蒙变化是更年期。在女性中使用荷尔蒙替代疗法主要是用于治疗严重的更年期症状，并且被称为更年期荷尔蒙替代疗法。推荐的使用对象是健康的女性，没有禁忌症，也没有过度的心血管或乳腺癌风险，并且年龄小于 60 岁或在更年期开始后小于 10 年。但是，长期使用荷尔蒙替代疗法是不合适的[1]。荷尔蒙替代疗法可减少更年期症状，骨质流失，骨折，糖尿病，心血管疾病和全因死亡率。但是，荷尔蒙替代疗法有长期的副作用，包括增加患癌，心肌梗塞和脑中风的风险[2,3]。最近，已证明具有相同生物特性(bioidentical) 或天然(natural) 荷尔蒙是有效的，副作用少，改善了生活品质，满意度更高[4,5,6]。这些天然荷尔蒙可能是荷尔蒙替代疗法的首选方法。

对于男性而言，与年龄相关的荷尔蒙变化是男性更年期或睾丸荷尔蒙随着年龄的增长而逐渐下降。男性睾丸荷尔蒙替代疗法的益处包括增强性功能，骨骼密度，肌肉质量，身体状况，情绪，红血球形成，认知，生活品质和减少心血管疾病[7]。补充睾丸荷尔蒙可能会引起心血管事件，高凝血状态（例如脑中风，深静脉血栓形成），肝酶升高，肝衰竭和肝癌的风险。由于缺乏明显的获益证据，尚无足够证据支持老年男性荷尔蒙替代疗法[8]。脱氢表雄酮（dehydroepiandrosterone，DHEA）是类固醇生成的先驱物，由肾上腺分泌。它被代谢成雄烯二酮，而雄烯二酮又被代谢成女性的雌酮和雌二醇，及代谢成男性的睾丸荷尔蒙。DHEA 引起了人们的兴趣，它是一种逆转与年龄相关的男性荷尔蒙缺乏的疗法。但是，尚未发现 DHEA 能显著逆转老化的功效[9]。

生长激素和类胰岛素生长因子随着衰老而下降，导致新陈代谢疾病，心血管变化和虚弱[10]。补充生长激素的好处包括提升生活品质，身体状况，肌肉力量，骨质密度，脂质增生，及减少心血管和脑血管发病率和死亡率[11]。临床研究已经评估了生长激素对于年龄相关的病变多个方面的作用，但尚未发现任何

益处[12]。

  总体而言，由于缺乏评估益处，风险和长期效果的临床研究，荷尔蒙替代疗法在抗衰老适应症中的应用受到限制[13]。

参考文献

1. Stuenkel CA, Davis SR, Gompel A et al. Treatment of symptoms of the menopause: an endocrine society clinical practice guideline. J Clin Endocrinol Meta 2015;100:3975-4011
2. Rossouw JE, Anderson GL, Prentice RL et al. Risks and benefits of estrogen plus progestin in healthy postmenopausal women: principal results from the women's health initiative randomized controlled trial. JAMA 2002;17:321-33
3. Chlebowski RT, Anderson LG, Gass MD et al. Estrogen plus progestin and breast cancer incidence and mortality in postmenopausal women. JAMA 2010;304:1684-90
4. Fitzpatrick LA, Pace C, Wiiter B. Comparison of regimens containing oral micronized progesterone of medroxyprogesterone acetate on quality of life in postmenopausal women: a cross-sectional survey. J Women Health Gend Based Med 200;9:38107
5. Hargrove JT, Maxson WS, Wentz AC et al. Menopausal hormone replacement therapy with continuous daily oral micronized progesterone. Obstet Gynecol 1989;73:606-12
6. Riis BJ, ThrmsenK, Strom V et al. The effect of percutaneous estradiol and natural progesterone on postmenopausal bone loss. Am J Obstet Gynecol 1987;156:61-5
7. Bassil N, Alkaade S, Morley JE. The benefits and risks of testosterone replacement therapy: a review. Ther Clin Risk Manag 2009;5(3):427-48
8. Schwartz E, Morelli V, Hottorf K. Hormone replacement therapy in the geriatric patient: current state of the evidence and questions for the future-estrogen, progesterone, testosterone and thyroid hormone augmentation in geriatric clinical practice: part 2. Clin Geriatr Med 2011;27:561-75
9. Legrain S, Girard L. Pharmacology and therapeutic effects of

dehydroepiandrosterone in older subjects. Drugs Aging 2003;20:949-67

10. Giaunoulis MF, Martin FC, Nair KS et al. Hormone replacement therapy and physical function in healthy older men. Time to talk hormones? Endocr Rev 2012;33:314-77
11. Carroll PV, Christ ER, Bengstsson BA et al. Growth hormone deficiency in adulthood and the effects of growth hormone replacement: a review. J Clin Endocrinol Metab 1998;83(2):382-95
12. Liu H, Brarada DM, Olkia I et al. Systematic review: the safety and efficacy of growth hormone in the healthy elderly. Ann Intern Med 2007;146:104-15
13. Samaras N, Papadopoulou MA, Samaras D et al. Off-label use of hormones as an antiaging strategy: a review. Clin Interv Aging 2014;9:1175-86

2.12 抗氧化剂

大气中氧气的存在是生命的决定因素，因为它提供生命所需的能量三磷酸腺苷 (adenosine triphosphate, ATP)。由于所有有氧生物在细胞呼吸和正常新陈代谢过程中都会利用氧气，因此通过生化细胞反应以及细胞呼吸（粒线体电子传输链, mitochondrial electron transport chain）产生活性氧（reactive oxygenspecies, ROS）是不可避免的[1]。此外，ROS 亦可从外界的污染物、烟草、烟雾、毒品、辐射和其他介质产生。在疾病和治疗过程中还会产生额外数量的 ROS。在生物系统中形成的含氧自由基分子及其先驱物统称为 ROS，是具有高反应性的分子，主要包括超氧化物，过氧化氢和羟基自由基。由于氧化作用是生命的基础，因此有必要在体内氧化和抗氧化防御之间保持适当的平衡。氧化压迫 (oxidative stress) 是由于过度氧化和/或缺乏抗氧化防御作用引起的。氧化压迫会严重破坏 DNA，蛋白质，脂质等分子，因此会导致多种疾病，如衰老、糖尿病、心血管和神经退化性疾病、癌症[2]。另一方面，氧化压迫可能是抵抗细菌或病毒的防御机制，在这种情况下，氧化压迫是一种保护机制。若用抗氧化剂阻止

该氧化压迫保护机制时，可能出现严重的临床问题。某些种类的细菌或癌细胞是通过有效的抗氧化系统保护自己。此外，ROS 是促进健康和长寿所必需的信号传导（诱导）分子。ROS 是骨骼肌肉正常力量产生，耐力表现发展以及人体防御系统诱导所必需的。很多生理功能是受到氧化还原（redox, 氧化压迫和抗氧化剂）信号通路机转的控制[3]，包括基因表达，新陈代谢调节，炎症反应，干细胞增殖和分化，癌症形成和衰老等[4,5]。生理量的 ROS 能诱发各种细胞功能，包括信号转导途径 (signal transduction pathways)，自噬机能 (autophagy，细胞清除细胞废弃物的机转以维持细胞等穩性)，细胞增生和凋亡（apoptosis，即程序性细胞死亡）[6]。此外，一旦抗氧化剂将其电子或氢原子提供给另一种物质，它就会成为一种「氧化剂」，能够从刚刚提供的另一种物质中获得电子或氢原子。换句话说，每种抗氧化剂都可以变成助氧化剂。因此，ROS 扮演着对生命系统有害或有益的双重角色。当 ROS 水平超出生理水平范围时，不管过低或过高，都会对健康产生不利影响。有氧生物已产生综合性良好的抗氧化防御能力。天然抗氧化剂是清除 ROS 的细胞防御机制，可以分为内源性（人体）抗氧化剂，天然和合成抗氧化剂。内源性抗氧化剂包括 glutathione, alpha-lipoid acid, coenzyme Q, ferritin, bilirubin, metallothionein, L-carnitine 及抗氧化酶如 catalase, superoxide dismutase 及 glutathione peroxidase。 天然抗氧化剂包括维生素 C，E 和 A，lipoic acid, glutathione 及 polyphenol metabolites。 合成抗氧化剂的例子包括 N-acetyl cysteine, tiron, pyrurate, selenium 等[7]。 在水果、蔬菜、坚果、油和种子等中发现了饮食中的抗氧化剂，例如维生素 A，C 和 E。 抗氧化剂与 ROS 反应，从而中和其化学活性。 抗氧化剂可以充当氧化剂的清除剂，以维持生物氧化还原等稳性。 ROS 与多种疾病有关，包括心血管和神经退化性疾病，肺和肾脏疾病，衰老和癌症[8]。 总体而言，缺乏证据表明抗氧化维生素对预防疾病有益。

与不食用维生素的人相比，经常食用抗氧化维生素 A 和 E 和 β-胡萝卜素等的人的死亡风险略高，并且没有证据支持抗氧化剂在预防和治疗衰老和疾病中的作用[9,10]。 此外，高剂量的维生素 C 和 E 降低了运动对人类受试者胰岛素敏感性和 ROS 水平的有益作用[11]。 迄今为止，已经有许多抗氧化剂疗法的临床试验。但是，这些抗氧化剂疗法的预防或治疗作用方面

结果大多是负面的[12]。尽管 ROS 可能通过诱导细胞损伤而导致衰老和疾病，但它们在细胞信号通路中也起着重要的作用，而用高剂量的抗氧化剂阻断其作用不一定能改善健康和寿命。在疾病状态下抗氧化剂治疗的目标，主要是使 ROS 水平升高恢复正常，并限制氧化损伤，而不是干扰 ROS 的正常生理作用。迄今为止，关于最佳生物分子指标用以测量体内氧化压迫尚无共识。由于 ROS 也具有有益的性质，因此仍然难以确定从生理性疾病到病理性疾病的氧化损伤引起的生物分子指标最佳范围，即对健康有害或有益的水平。建立抗氧化剂的最佳滴定剂量还需要进一步的研究。氧化还原平衡 (redox balance) 应严格控制，因为 ROS 的缺乏和过量都会引起病理和疾病。

参考文献

1. Lushchak VI. Free radicals, reactive oxygen species, oxidative stress and its classification. Chem Biol Interact 2014;224:164-75
2. Reuter S, Gupta SC, Chaturvedi MM, Aggarwal BB. Oxidative stress, inflammation and cancer: how are they linked? Free Rad Biol Med 2010;49(11):1603-16
3. Wu P et al. FDA-approved small-molecule kinase inhibitors. Trends Pharmacol Sci 2015;36:L422-39
4. Holmstrom KM, Finkel T. Cellular mechanisms and physiological consequences of redox-dependent signaling. Nat Rev Mol Cell Biol 2014;15:411
5. Schieber M, Chandel NS. ROS function in redox signaling and oxidative stress. Curr Biol 2014;24:R453-R462
6. Jisun L, Samantha G, Jianhua Z. Autophagy, mitochondria and oxidative stress: cross-talk and redox signaling. Biochem J 2012;441(2):523-40
7. Yoshida T, Oka S, Masutani H, Nakamnra HG, Yodoi J. The role of thioredoxin in the aging process: involvement of oxidative stress. Antioxidants Redox Signaling 2003;5:563-70
8. Halliwell B, Gutteridge JMC. Free radicals in biology and medicine (4th ed), Oxford University Press, 2007.
9. Bjelakovic G, Nikolova D, Gluud LL, Simonetti RB, Gluud C. Mortality in randomized trials of antioxidant supplements for primary and secondary prevention: systematic review and meta-analysis. JAMA 2007;297:842-57
10. Bjelakovic G et al. Antioxidant supplement for prevention of mortality in healthy participants and patients with various diseases. Cochrane Database Syst Rev 2013;

CD007176
11. Ristow M et al. Antioxidants prevent health-promoting effects of physical exercise in humans. Proc Natl Acad Sci USA 2009;106:8665-8670
12. Steinhubl SR. Why have antioxidants failed in clinical trials? Am J Cardiol 2008;101(10A):14D-19D

2.13 另类医学

许多人在正规医学之外寻找至少一部分另类医疗保健。另类医学 (alternative medicine) 是指正规医学院没有实行的医学方法。补充医学 (complementary medicine) 是指使用另类医学作为常规医学的辅助手段。将另类医学和补充医学整合到正规医学实践中的方法称为整合医学 (integrative medicine)。

维生素和其他微量营养素

正常人体功能需要微量的维生素和矿物质。但是，「越多越好」的概念，即由于摄入不足，吸收不良或组织需求增加而导致的某些缺乏状态下，摄入超出建议的每日摄入量 (recommended daily allowances) 的维生素和矿物质，被怀疑是无益的，并且在某些情况下可能是有害的。正分子医学 (orthomolecular medicine) 是通过补充营养来恢复和维持健康，例如维生素，矿物质，氨基酸，微量元素和脂肪酸。高剂量的营养素具有预防和治疗作用。维生素 C 和 E，β-胡萝卜素，B 族复合维生素，矿物质

、必需脂肪酸，氨基酸，植物化学物质，辅酶 Q10 和辅助食品因子是许多改善营养和长寿的营养素，其剂量远高于建议的每日摄入量 (recommended daily allowances)。

通常，对于大多数实行健康饮食的人来说，不需要补充维生素。高剂量的维生素，尤其是脂溶性维生素具有风险和毒性。正分子医学背后的观点没有医学证据的支持，并且该疗法无效。

辅酶 Q10 (coenzyme Q10) 存在于大多数食品中，尤其是肉和鱼。辅酶 Q10 也因其在自然界中的普遍分布而被称为泛醌 (ubiquinone)，它是一种抗氧化剂，也是粒线体呼吸链中不可或缺的组成部分，可产生能量。它存在于人体的所有组织和器官中，但在心脏中的浓度最高。随着衰老和心血管疾病（例如高血压和心脏衰竭），辅酶 Q10 水平下降。辅酶 Q10 对心肌至关重要，它有助于降低血压，改善缺血性心脏病和心脏衰竭，并在退化性脑疾病中保护大脑[1]。辅酶 Q10 具有抗氧化和抗炎活性，可改善血管内皮功能[2]。

尽管有许多益处的声明，但仍需要进行有关辅酶 Q10 剂量和功效的进一步临床研究。尽管如此，由于临床研究规模相对较小，补充辅酶 Q10 的证据仍然只是中等水平。

左旋肉碱 (L-carnitine) 是一种主要由氨基酸 lysine 及 methionine 合成的氨基酸衍生物，在脂肪酸代谢中起作用。左旋肉碱通常存在于红肉和乳制品中，例如牛奶和奶酪。左旋肉碱是一种具有多种生理功能的天然物质，可能有效治疗各种心血管疾病。小型研究表示，左旋肉碱饮食补充剂对心肌梗塞后心脏重塑[3]，运动能力[4]，改善心脏射血分数（ejection fraction, 心脏收缩力）和心脏衰竭患者的临床结果有益[5,6]。在可以提出建议之前，还需要对这种物质进行进一步的临床研究。左旋精氨酸 (L-arginine) 是人体必需的氨基酸，可作为一氧化氮生产的前驱物。左旋精氨酸可增强人和实验动物中血管内皮一氧化氮的产生[7,8]。左旋精氨酸对血管内皮，免疫系统具有有益作用，并调节肿瘤的生长和增殖[9,10]。

一氧化氮 (nitric oxide) 是一种重要的多能的气态细胞信号传导 (诱导) 分子。它是通过左旋精氨酸—

氧化氮合酶途径 (L-arginine-nitric oxide synthases pathway) 在体内产生的，或者是从饮食中摄入的硝酸盐、亚硝酸盐通过硝酸盐、亚硝酸盐及一氧化氮途径 (nitrate-nitrite-nitric oxide pathway) 产生。一氧化氮可导致血管舒张并降低血压，减少炎症，降低血管通透性，减少低密度脂蛋白氧化 (坏胆固醇作用) 并抑制血管平滑肌增殖[11,12]。一氧化氮在调节血管张力[13]，神经传递[14]和免疫系统中起作用[15]。一氧化氮还是粒线体形成的调节剂。粒线体功能受损与神经退化性疾病，神经肌肉疾病，肝和心脏衰竭，糖尿病有关[16,17]。

氨基酸混合物 (amino acid mixtures) 在心脏新陈代谢中起作用。它们是蛋白质的组成部分，是能量新陈代谢的中间代谢物[18]。已经提出将它们用作治疗心脏衰竭和糖尿病的方法。补充氨基酸会诱导蛋白质合成并增加肌肉质量和功能[19]。氨基酸是大脑神经传导递质的前驱物，包括 serotonin, dopamine, norepinephrine, 与情绪和行为有关[20]。氨基酸可改善瘦体重，强度和身体机能以及日常生活活动[21]。此外，已指出由 isoleucine, cystine, methionine, valine 及 leucine 组成的氨基酸混合物可改善糖尿病

患者对血糖的控制[22]。

膳食酶补充剂(dietary enzyme supplements)，例如菠萝蛋白酶(bromelain)，木瓜蛋白酶(papain)，胰蛋白酶(trypsin)和胰凝乳蛋白酶(chymotrypsin)，以及多种组合产品，已上市销售，并宣称能有效改善健康并治疗炎性疾病，过敏，伤口，烧伤，感染，骨关节炎，肌肉酸痛，胃肠道症状，多发性硬化症，胰腺功能不全和癌症。然而，缺乏支持膳食酶补充的证据，需要更大的研究来评估其有益效果。

总体而言，目前各种补充剂有益健康的临床数据或证据有限。

心身方法

压力会通过造成身心系统的不平衡而加剧疾病。压力可能会对儿茶酚胺(catecholamine)和皮质醇(cortisol)水平，葡萄糖代谢，自主神经和血管紧张，凝血，疼痛感和免疫功能产生不利影响。心身方

法可以减轻压力，包括放松和锻炼技巧，例如冥想和祈祷，瑜伽，太极拳，气功，音乐疗法，幽默和笑声，芳香疗法，催眠，行为改变，生物反馈和使用引导性想像。

瑜伽有多种技巧，包括冥想，放松，伸展和控制呼吸，以达到放松和健身的状态。瑜伽是印度草药疗法 (Ayurvedic medicine) 的主要项目，这是印度古代的整体保健方法，重点在于瑜伽，冥想，饮食，药用植物和其他疗法。

芳香疗法被定义为吸入香气以产生治疗效果。已经显示出令人愉悦的香气会影响血压，心律，凝血和放松作用。

生物反馈 (biofeedback) 是一种身心疗法，通常与放松训练相结合，作为对压力相关疾病的治疗。生物反馈包括监视和显示有关生理功能的信息，例如心率，脑电波，肌电图和热能反应。利用这些生物反馈信息，可以进行诸如深呼吸，冥想和想像之类的放松技能。

引导想像 (guided imagery) 是一种放松的，集中的状态，通过引导想像力并使用指导思想和建议来实行，从而产生所需的生理和社会心理效果。引导想像可以减轻压力，提高免疫和心血管功能。

光生物调节

光生物调节 (photobiomodulation) 是用低强度的红色至近红外激光（600-1100 nm）照射细胞或组织，以治愈，恢复和刺激多个生理过程以及修复由疾病或创伤引起的损害。光疗法的生物效应是将光能量转化为新陈代谢能量，从而调节细胞功能[23,24]。现在光生物调节的临床应用包括口腔粘膜的组织和伤口愈合（口腔粘膜发炎）[25]，糖尿病足溃疡[26]和软组织损伤[27]，缓解疼痛，中风，心肌梗塞，关节炎，衰老，癌症和退化性或外伤性脑疾病[28,29,30]。在心肌损伤和神经退化性疾病的情况下，局部光生物调节可以增强远处，未照射的组织的等隐性，这种现象称为间接光生物调节[31]。光生物调节似乎为保护重要的器官（如脑，心脏和肾脏）免受缺血和疾病的压力提供了一种安全且无侵入性的治疗选择。光生物调节仍存在争议，因为其在分子，细胞和组织水平上的作用机转

尚不确定。此外，很多的参数（例如波长，能量密度，辐照度，治疗时间和重复性，脉冲和极化）是随意性的，并且存在双相剂量效应，即低剂量可获得益处，而高剂量则有害。

量子医学

量子医学 (quantum medicine) 基于医学，量子物理学，生物物理学，电子学和生物共振的知识。身体的每个细胞代表一个电磁单元，该电磁单元发出理想频率的特定电磁波。当理想的电磁波频率由于外部和内部因素而改变时，生化过程就会发生变化，从而导致疾病的形成。量子医学领域最强大的设备是用于诊断目的的生物共振 (bioresonance) 和热成像扫描仪 (thermovision scanner)，以及用于治疗目的的微共振(microresonance) 和 Rikta 治疗。诊断扫描仪可以检测电磁场的变化，从而得出有关某些器官和组织功能受损以及是否为炎症，退化，良性或可疑恶性病变的结论。微共振和 Rikta 治疗向人体施加了几种类型的生物刺激性电磁辐射，它们强度低且安全，可以使疾病中受干扰的磁场恢复正常。

参考文献

1. Janson M. Orthomolecular medicine: the therapeutic use of dietary supplements for antiaging. Clin Interventions Aging 2006;1(3):261-5
2. Pepe S, Marasco SF, Haas SJ et al. Coenzyme Q10 in cardiovascular disease. Mitochondrion 2007;7 supp: S154
3. Iliceto S, Scrutinio D, Bruzzi P et al. Effects of L-carnitine administration on left ventricular remodeling after acute myocardial infarction: the L-carnitine echocardogratia digitalizzata infarto miocardico (CEDIM) trial. J Am Coll Cardiol 1995;26:380-7
4. Anand IS, Francis G, Maseri A et al. Study on propionyl-l-carnitine in chronic heart failure. Eur Heart J 1999;20:70-6
5. Anand I, Chandrashekhan Y, De Gluli F et al. Acute and chronic effects of propionyl-l-carnitine on the hemodynamics, exercise capacity, and hormone in patients with congestive heart failure. Cardiovasc Drug Ther 1998;12:291-9
6. Rizos I. Three-year survival of patients with heart failure caused by dilated cardiomyopathy and L-carnitine administration. Am Heart J 2000;139:S20-3
7. Hishikawa K, Nakak T, Tsuda M et al. Effect of systemic L-arginine administration on hemodynamic and nitric oxide release in man. Jpn Heart J 1992;33:41-8
8. Cernadas MR, Lopez-Farre A, Riesco A et al. Renal and systemic effects of aminoacids administration seperately: comparison between L-arginine and non-nitric oxide donor aminoacids. J Pharmacol Exp Ther 1992;263:1023-9
9. Albina JE, Caldwell MD, Henry Jr WL, Mills CD. Regulation of macrophage functions by L-arginine. J Exp Med 1989;169:1021-9
10. Brittenden J, Heys SD, Eremin O. L-arginine and malignant disease: a potential therapeutic role? Eur J Surg Oncol 1994;20:189-92

11. Lundberg JO, Weitzberg E, Gladwin MT. The nitrate-nitrite-nitric oxide pathway in physiology and therapeutics. Nat Rev Drug Discov 2008;7:156-67
12. Li H, Horke S, Forstermann U. Vascular oxidative stress, nitric oxide and atherosclerosis. Atherosclerosis 2014;237:208-19
13. Palmer RMJ, Ferrige AG, Moncada S. Nitric oxide release accounts for the biological activity of endothelium-derived relaxing factor. Nature 1987;327:524-6
14. Knowles RG, Palacios M, Palmer RMJ, Moncada S. Formation of nitric oxide from L-arginine in the central nervous system: a transduction mechanism for stimulation of soluble guanylate cyclase. Proc Natl Acad Sci USA 1989;86:5159-62
15. Hibbs JB Jr, Taintor R, Vavrin Z, Rachlin EM. Nitric oxide: a cytotoxic activated macrophage effector molecule. Biochem Biophys Res Commun 1988;157:87-94
16. Hansford RG, Tsuchiya N, Pepe S. Mitochondria in heart ischemia and aging. Biochem Soc Symp 1999;66:141-7
17. Patti ME, Butte AJ, Crunkhorn S et al. Coordinated reduction of genes of oxidative metabolism in humans with insulin resistance and diabetes: potential role of PGC1 and NRF1. Proc Natl Acad Sci USA 2003;100:8466-71
18. Taegtmeyer H, Harinstein ME, Gheorghiade M. More than bricks and mortar: comments on protein and amino acid metabolism in the heart. Am J Cardiol 2008;101:3E-7E
19. Aquilani R, Oposich C, Gualco A et al. Adequate energy-protein intake is not enough to improve nutritional and metabolic status in muscle-depleted patients with chronic heart failure. Eur J Heart Fail 2008;10:1127-35
20. Fernstrom JD, Faller DV. Neutral amino acids in the brain: changes in response to food ingestion. J Neurochem 1978;30:1531-8
21. Walrand S, Boirie Y. Optimizing protein intake in aging.

Curr Opin Clin Nutr Metab Care 2005;8:89-94
22. Wang B, Kammer LM, Ding Z et al. Amino acid mixture acutely improves the glucose tolerance of healthy overweight adults. Nutr Res 2012;32:30-8
23. Hashmi JT. Role of low-level laser therapy in neurorehabilitation. PMR 2010;2:S292-305
24. Khan I, Arany P. Biophysical approaches for oral wound healing: emphasis on photobiomodulation. Adv Wound Care 2015;4(12):724-37
25. Fekrazad R, Chiniforush N. Oral mucositis prevention and management by therapeutic laser in head and neck cancers. Lasers Med Sci 2014;5:1-7
26. Tchanque-Fossuo CN, Ho D, Dahle SE et al. A systemic review of low-level light therapy for treatment of diabetic foot ulcer. Wound Repair Regen 2016;24:418-26
27. Bjordal JM, Johnson MI, Iversen V, Aimbire F, Lopers-Martins RG. Low-level laser therapy in acute pain : a systemic review of possible mechanisms of action and clinical effects in randomized placebo-controlled trials. Photomed Laser Surg 2006;24:158-68
28. Blatt A, Elbaz-Greener GA, Tuby H et al. Low-level laser therapy to the bone marrow reduces scarring and improves heart function post-acute myocardial infarction in the pig. Photomed laser Surg 2016;34:516-24
29. Farfara D, Tuby H, Trudler D et al. Low-level laser therapy ameliorates disease progression in a mouse model of Alzheimer's disease. J Mol Neurosci 2005;55:430-6
30. Johnstone DM, Massri N, Moro C et al. Indirect application of near infrared light induces neuroprotection in a mouse model of parkinsonism – an abscopal neuroprotective effect. Neurosci 2014;274:93-101
31. Kim B, Brandli A, Mitrofauis J et al. Remote tissue conditioning – an emerging approach for inducing body-wide protection against disease of aging. Aging Research Review 2017;37:69-78

老化

第三章

老化及抗老化

3.1 老化

老化有两个主要部分。按年代的老化 (chronological aging) 是指人的实际年龄，以年，月和日为单位，这是不可停止，不可改变且不可逆的。生理或生物老化 (physiological or biological aging) 是根据个体某些细胞或分子参数的发展和变化而定。生理老化是随着年代的老化推移引发健康恶化并最终导致死亡的一系列过程，是可以逆转或延长的[1,2]。由于老化(aging) 伴随着细胞，组织，器官和体内系统正常生理功能的损害，会增加身体疾病和死亡风险，老化被认为是致命的疾病[3,4]。的确，老化是一个复杂的过程，其特征是身体，精神和生殖能力逐渐下降，导致功能丧失，增加身体疾病并最后终止生命。老化是慢性疾病和残疾状况的主要危险因素，包括心脏病，癌症，中风，慢性阻塞性肺疾病，慢性肾脏病，糖尿病，老人痴呆。毫无疑问，老化是身体结构和功能的有害异常，并且老化还具有特定的原因以及可识别的体征和症状。老化领域的当前挑战是缺乏用于测量老化的标准参数。老化是所有老年相关疾病的总和，而且这是老化的最佳生物指标。预防医学的目的是通过治疗未病来预防将病。因此，预防医学可以被认为是

抗衰老疗法的一种方案。预防医学和抗衰老疗法都是通过治疗健康个体来预防未病。预防医学药物中使用的某些药物，例如 statins，aspirin，可以重新用作抗衰老药物。抗衰老医疗是减少晚年疾病的任何预防方法。

老化的特征是生理机能的逐渐丧失，导致身体功能，发病率和死亡率恶化。这种恶化导致癌症，心血管疾病，糖尿病和神经退化性疾病。随着时间的推移，细胞损伤的累积是老化的普遍原因。最近概述了九个「老化标志」("hallmarks of aging")：基因组不稳定 (genomic instability)，端粒（telomere,染色体末端）磨损，基因外改变 (epigenetic alteration)，蛋白质稳性（proteostasis）丧失，营养调节 (nutrient-sensing) 失调，粒线体 (mitochondria) 功能障碍，细胞衰老 (cellular senescence)，干细胞耗尽，及细胞间的交流改变 (intercellular communication)[5]。

基因组不稳定是一生中遗传损伤的累积。一些染色体区域，例如端粒，特别容易受到与年老相关的损害和退化的影响，从而导致端粒丢失和缩短（端粒磨损），细胞衰老和身体衰老。老化伴随着基因外改

变导致染色体改变，称为外基因改变。老化与受损的蛋白质稳性有关。蛋白质稳性丧失会导致蛋白质的展开，折叠或聚集，从而导致老年相关的疾病。细胞生长需要营养和营养物质可用性的准确信号传递。营养信号传递感应失控会导致老化。随着年龄的增长而发生的粒线体功能障碍导致自由基（reactive oxidative species, ROS）的产生增加，进而导致粒线体进一步恶化和损伤。细胞衰老是细胞周期的稳定停滞(arrest of cell cycle，所以细胞停止分化、发展)，导致身体衰老。干细胞耗尽是组织再生潜能的下降，导致衰老。例如，血液的形成随着年龄的增长而下降，导致免疫细胞的产生减少，从而导致贫血和血癌的发生率增加。衰老还涉及细胞间交流改变(intercellular communication)，例如内分泌，神经内分泌或神经元介体(neuronal mediators)。

在世界范围内，众所周知，人口正在老龄化。65岁以上老人中有70%以上患有两种或更多种慢性疾病，例如关节炎，糖尿病，癌症，心脏病和脑中风[6]。人口老龄化的主要挑战是维持身体和认知功能，生活质量和独立性。老化是一个持续的过程，其中包括功能丧失和取决于众多遗传，环境和生活方式因素的

变化。老年人的生理储备明显减少，导致无法耐受压迫以恢复其体内等稳性。

大多数器官，组织和细胞逐渐老化，效率降低。同一人的器官系统以不同的速度老化。65 岁以后，大脑的体积会减少，并且脑血流量也会减少。与年老引起的脑细胞损失很可能是由于凋亡（apoptosis，即程序性细胞死亡）引起的，而不是炎症，局部缺血或其他机制引起的[7]。随着年龄的增长，脑酶（brain enzymes），受体（brain receptors）和神经递质(neurotransmitters) 会发生多种非均质变化。老化与大脑下丘脑-垂体-肾上腺轴区域失调，神经传递(neurotransmission) 和神经营养因子 (neurotrophic factor) 信号传导（诱导）失调，炎性状态增加，基因和外基因变化，氧化压迫，新陈代谢变化以及肠微生态-脑轴 (microbiota-gut-brain axis) 相互关系改变有关。这些机制导致大脑适应可塑性改变，免疫系统失调，大脑功能下降以及罹患脑部疾病的风险增加。眼睛的结构随年龄而变化。眼睛周边组织萎缩，眼睑变得更加松弛。泪腺功能，泪液产生和杯状细胞 (goblet cell, 分泌黏液) 功能均降低。结膜萎缩和变黄。角膜中胆固醇酯，胆固醇和中性脂肪的沉积会引

起 arcus senilis，这是在角膜周围的环状黄白色沉淀物。 晶状体(lens) 和虹膜 (iris) 的改变导致老花眼。由于晶状体弹性降低，并且在较小程度上眼睫状肌减弱和丧失有效角度，聚焦在近物所需的距离增加[8]。年老相关的听力系统变化会导致听力下降。 随着年龄的增长，外耳道壁变薄。耳垢变得更干燥和更黏稠，老年人耳垢阻塞耳道的发生率增加。 老年相关的味觉和嗅觉下降可能会导致食物和营养缺乏症。

老化是心血管疾病风险的主要决定因素。 其主要原因是过度的氧化压迫和慢性低度发炎，添加在有限的心脏再生能力上[9]。 年龄增长会增加患高血压和冠心病的风险。血管内皮衰老会提高血管壁的硬度，导致更高的收缩压和脉压。 血管交感神经受体不感应，导致姿势性低血压的趋势增加。 随着年龄的增长，左心房增大，左心室变僵硬和肥大[10]。 还有心脏细胞肥大和损失[11]。 心脏主动脉和二尖瓣均增厚并钙化[12]。 心率改变性 (heart rate variability, 心率调节功能) 也随年龄增长而降低，可能由于副交感神经张力降低和交感神经反应下降所致[13]。 心脏心律不整的发生率随年龄增长而增加[14]。 老化与心脏纤维化的产生有关，导致心脏衰竭[15]。

呼吸系统中与年龄相关的解剖和功能变化导致老年人慢性肺部疾病，肺炎，缺氧和氧吸收减少。肺部发生解剖变化。肺泡管增大，导致交换气体的表面积减小，肺部非气体交换空间亦增加，导致气体扩散能力降低。老化增加了气体通气-灌注不配合，因为在呼吸周期中，比其他地方更好灌注的老年肺中依赖部分的气道关闭，导致氧饱和度随年龄下降。胸壁增加僵硬度。横隔膜变平，功能降低。肺功能储备和肺功能下降。在老年人中，咳嗽的强度较小，粘液清除的速度较慢，效果较差。

老化对胃肠系统的总体影响是适度的。老化本身不会引起营养不良。口腔粘膜随着年龄的增长而变薄。牙龈萎缩，露出牙骨质，牙骨质更容易腐烂，使老年人容易患上龋齿，咀嚼不完全以及营养摄入不足的危险[16,17]。多达50%的老年人抱怨口干，可能会影响咀嚼和吞咽，这可能是由于与老化相关的唾液分泌减少所致[18]。老年人胃炎的发生率增加可能与若干老化相关的生理变化有关：前列腺素的合成减少，bicarbonate 和非顶壁液 (nonparietal fluid) 的分泌减少，胃排空延迟和微循环障碍[19]。胃还具有内分泌功能。老年人的血清 ghrelin 和 gastrin 激素水平降

低[20]。小肠亦有中等程度的绒毛萎缩和粘膜变粗。微量营养素和一般营养素的吸收会随着年龄的增长而减少，但仍足以保持体内等稳性[21]。大肠有黏膜萎缩，细胞和结构异常，结肠推进动力减少。结肠癌的风险随着年龄的增长而增加。除了长时间暴露于潜在的致癌物外，老化还与结肠粘膜增生和凋亡（apoptosis，即程序性细胞死亡）减少有关[22]。肝质量，肝灌流和血流量随年龄的增长而降低[23]。然而，标准的肝功能测试随年龄的增长而受到的影响很小[24]。尽管胆囊的功能和解剖结构在老年人中保存得很好，但胆汁成分具有很高的生石作用（结石指数），使老年人容易产生胆结石[25]。

随着年龄的增长，功能性肾小球（glomeruli，肾脏的动脉单位），肾脏血浆流量，肾脏质量和整体肾脏功能会降低。在大多数临床研究中，由于肾单位（nephron，肾脏的解剖和功能单位）的丧失，肾小球滤过率（glomerular filtration rate，GFR）的平均损失约为每年 1 ml[26]。随着年龄的增长，还会发生各种结构变化，包括微解剖学变化，例如肾硬化和肾单位数目的减少，以及一般解剖学变化，例如肾脏体积的减少，肾动脉的动脉粥样硬化和肾囊肿的产生。

热量限制 (节食，calorie restriction) 可以预防或延迟与老化相关的肾脏病变的发生[26]。肾脏的荷尔蒙功能也受到老化的影响，包括维生素 D 产量下降和肾素-血管紧张素-醛固酮 (rennin-angiotensin-aldosterone system) 神经激素系统的下调。在没有压迫的情况下，随着老化，流体和电解质的动态平衡保持相对良好。

泌尿生殖系统的老化增加了老年人尿失禁，尿路感染，勃起功能障碍和女性性交困难或疼痛的风险。尿失禁与膀胱肌肉收缩力降低、最大膀胱容量、最大尿流速和抑制排尿的能力有关，并伴有余尿的增加[27]。随着年龄的增长，前列腺也会增大。

与年老有关的肌肉质量和力量的丧失，以及脂肪质量的增加，导致运动和平衡受损，虚弱和身体机能下降。年老的肌肉也更容易疲劳。生长激素，雄激素等的老化相关激素变化可能与肌肉质量和功能的变化有关。一旦发生骨折，老年人的骨折发生率较高，修复速度减慢。骨质下降，维生素 D 缺乏症（老年人常见）进一步加剧了骨质流失。

在没有其他压迫的情况下，造血（血液形成）系统在整个人的一生中都可以维持适当的功能[28]。红血细胞的寿命，铁质的更替率和血容量不会随着年龄的增长而变化[29]。但是，随着年龄的增长，骨髓的质量会下降，骨髓中的脂肪也会增加。造血功能储备会随着年龄的增长而减少。老年人对缺氧，失血和其他压迫的代偿性造血反应会被延长并且效能降低[30]。这是由于先驱细胞群(progenitor cells)的变化以及骨髓环境基质(matrix，因子)的变化所致[31]。老化伴随着衰老的造血系统包括：免疫系统受损，自体免疫疾病，血液系统癌症和与老年相关的贫血的发生率增加。尽管血小板的数量不随年龄而变化，但血小板对许多血栓刺激物例如一氧化氮的减少和氧化损伤的增加会反应过度[32]。此外，老年人的血纤蛋白原(fibrinogen)，5、7、8、9因子，高分子量激肽原，前激肽释放酶，纤溶酶原激活物抑制剂-1（plasminogen activator inhibitor，血纤蛋白溶解的主要抑制剂），血纤蛋白降解片段（fibrin degradation fragments，D-dimers）升高[33,34,35]。因此，应将老年视为促凝状态(procoagulant state)，并且年龄是血栓形成的重要危险因素。血流淤滞(blood flow stasis)是血栓形成发生的重要因素，

在老年人中更常见。 年龄与动脉僵硬度的增加和血液动力学的改变相关，从而导致血管内皮功能障碍，进而导致血小板活化，聚集和血栓形成 [36]。

皮肤的正常老化会导致萎缩，弹性下降以及新陈代谢和修复反应受损。皮肤的感官知觉下降，尤其是在下肢 [37]。 皮下脂肪减少。 这种支撑的丧失会导致皮肤起皱和下垂，并增加对创伤的可能性 [38]。

所有的免疫细胞都起源于骨髓中的造血干细胞，随着年龄的增长，骨髓的造血组织普遍减少。 因老化而下降的免疫功能导致感染，癌症和自体免疫性疾病的发生增加 [39]。 免疫系统分为先天免疫 (innate immunity) 和适应性免疫 (adaptive immunity)。 先天免疫是指因暴露于微生物/抗原，从出生开始就存在的免疫反应，是不需学习或适应的。 先天免疫系统由上皮屏障（皮肤，胃肠道和呼吸道粘膜），巨噬细胞 (macrophage)，嗜中性粒细胞 (neutrophil)，天然杀伤细胞 (natural killer cell)，树突状细胞 (dendritic cell) 和补体蛋白 (complement) 组成。 适应性免疫由 T 和 B 淋巴细胞的细胞和体液（抗体）免疫反应组成，是由于个体一生中接触抗原所产生和适应的。 老

化既影响先天免疫又影响适应性免疫,尽管先天免疫机制总体上得到了更好的维持。在老年人中,T 和 B 细胞对抗原刺激的反应较小[40]。老年人经常出现全身性慢性低度炎症,这种炎症被称为「老化发炎」(inflammaging)[41]。衰老细胞产生促炎细胞因子(proinflammatory cytokines,IL-1、IL-6、IL-8)、肿瘤坏死因子(tumor necrosis factor,TNF)、C 反应蛋白(C-reactive protein,CRP)的水平升高,并且增加心血管和神经退化性疾病的风险,亦提升肌肉丧失、虚弱、总体发病率和死亡率[42]。

参考文献

1. Jia L, Zhang W, Chen X. Common methods of biological age estimation. Clin Interv Aging 2017;12:759-72
2. Booth LN, Brunet A. The aging epigenome. Mol Cell 2016;62:728-44
3. Bulterijs S, Hull RS, Bjork VC, Roy AG. It is time to classify biological aging as a disease. Front Genet 2015;6:205
4. Aunan JR, Wetson MM, Hagland HR, Soreide K. Molecular and biological hallmarks of aging. Br J Surg 2016;103:e29-46
5. Lopez-Otin C, Blasco MA, Partidge L, Serrano M, Kroemer G. The hallmarks of aging. Cell 2013;153(6):1194-1217
6. Hung WW, Ross JS, Boockvar KS, Siu AL. Recent trends in chronic disease, impairment and disability among older adults in the United States. BMC Geroatr 2011;11:47
7. Sastry PS, Rao KS. Apoptosis and the nervous system. J Neurochem 2000;74:1
8. Strenki SA, Strenk LM, Koretz JF. The mechanism of presbyopia. Prog Retin Eye Res 2005;24:379
9. LaKatta EG. Arterial and cardiac aging: major shareholders in cardiovascular disease enterprises part III: cellular and molecular clues to heart and arterial aging. Circulation 2003;107:490-7
10. Gates PE, Tanaka H, Graves J, Seals DR. Left ventricular structure and diastolic function with human aging. Relation to habitual exercise and arterial stiffness. Eur Heart J 2003;24:2213
11. Bergmann O, Bhardwaj RD, Bernard S et al. Evidence for cardiomyocyte renewal in humans. Science 2009;324:98
12. Kitzman DW, Scholz DG, Hagen PT et al. Age-related changes in normal human hearts during the first 10

decades of life. Part II (Maturity): A quantitative anatomic study of 765 specimens from subjects 20 to 99 years old. Mayo Clin Proc 1988;63:137
13. Parati G, Di Rienzo M. Determinants of heart rate and heart rate variability. J Hypertens 2003;21:477
14. Fleg JL, Kennedy HL. Long-term prognostic significance of ambulatory electrocardiographic findings in apparently healthy subjects greater than or equal to 60 years of age. Am J Cardiol 1992;70:748
15. Horu MA, Trafford AW. Aging and the cardiac collagen matrix: Novel mediators of fibrotic remodeling. J Mol Cell Cardiol 2016;93:175-85
16. Hall KE, Protor DD, Fisher L, Rose S. American gastroenterological association future trends committee report: effects of aging of the population on gastroenterology practice, education and research. Gastroenterology 2005;129:1305
17. Dunn-Walters DK, Howard WA, Bible JM. The aging gut. Mech Ageing Dev 2004;125:851
18. Smith CH, Boland B, Daureeawoo Y et al. Effect of aging on stimulated salivary flow in adults. J Am Geriatr Soc 2013;61:805
19. Guslandi M, Pellagrini A, Sorghi M. Gastric mucosal defences in the elderly. Gerontology 1999;45:206
20. Yin Y, Zhang W. The role of ghrelin in senescence: a mini-review. Gerontology 2016;62:155
21. Saltzman JR, Russell RM. The aging gut. Nutritional issues. Gastroenterol Clin North Am 1998;27:309
22. Xiao ZO, Moragoda L, Jaszewski R et al. Aging is associated with increased proliferation and decreased apoptosis in the colonic mucosa. Mech Ageing Dev 2001;122:1849
23. McLean AJ, Le Couteur DG. Aging biology and geriatric clinical pharmacology. Pharmacol Rev 2004;56:163
24. Rahmioglu N, Andrew T, Cherkas L et al. Epidemiology

and genetic epidemiology of the liver function test proteins. PLoS One 2009;4:e4435
25. Valdivieso V, Palma R, Wunkhaus R et al. Effect of aging on biliary lipid composition and bile acid metabolism in normal Chilean women. Gastroenterology 1978;74:871
26. Nadon NL. Of mice and monkeys: National Institute on aging resources supporting the use of animal models in biogerontology research. J Gerontol A Biol Sci Med Sci 2006;61(8):813-5
27. Elbadawi A, Diokno AC, Millard RJ. The aging bladder: morphology and urodynamics. World J Urol 1998;16 suppl 1: S10
28. Sansoni P, Cossarizza A, Brianti V et al. Lymphocyte subsets and natural killer cell activity in healthy old people and centenarians. Blood 1993;82:2767
29. Kirkland JL, Tchkonia T, Pirtskhalara T et al. Adipogenesis and aging: does aging make fat go mad? Exp Gerontol 2002;37:757
30. Boggs DR, Patrene KD. Hematopoiosis and aging III: Anemia and a blunted erythropoietic response to hemorrhage in aged mice. Am J Hematol 1985;19:P327
31. Albright JW, Makinodar T. Decline in the growth potential of spleen-colonizing bone marrow stem cells of long-lived aging mice. J Exp Med 1976;144:1204
32. Fuenter E, Palomo I. Role of oxidative stress on platelet hyperreactivity during aging. Life Sci 2016;148:17
33. Franchini M. Hemostasis and aging. Crit Rev Oncol Hematol 2006;60:144
34. Isaia G, Greppi F, Ausiello L et al. D-dimer plasma concentrations in an older hospitalized population. J Am Geriatr Soc 2011;59:2385
35. Mehta J, Mehta P, Lawson D, Saldeen T. Plasma tissue plasminogen activator inhibitor levels in coronary artery disease: correlation with age and serum triglycerides concentrations. J Am Coll Cardiol 1987;9:263

36. Thijssen DH, Carter SE, Green DJ. Arterial structure and function in vascular aging: are you as old as your arteries? J Physiol 2016;594:2275-84
37. Perry SD. Evaluation of age-related plantar-surface insensitivity and onset age of advanced insensitivity in older adults using vibratory and touch sensation tests. Neurosci Lett 2006;392:62
38. McCullough JL, Kelly KM. Prevention and treatment of skin aging. Ann NY Acad Sci 2006;1067:323
39. Geiger H, Rudolph KL. Aging in the lympho-hematopoietic stem cell compartment. Trends Immunol 2009;30:360
40. Weiskopf D, Weinberger B, Grubeck-Loebenstein B. The aging of the immune system. Transpl Int 2009;22:1041
41. Franceschi C, Campisi J. Chronic inflammation (inflammaging) and its potential contribution to age-associated disease. J Gerontol A Biol Sci Med Sci 2014;69(suppl 1):S4-9
42. Giuvita B et al. Inflammaging as a prodrome to Alzhemier's disease. J Neuroinflammation 2008;5:51

3.2 抗老化

疾病可以定义为结构或功能的失常或异常。一些人认为，老化不可能是异常的，因为每个人都会衰老，这导致人们不愿接受老化等同于疾病。延缓老化远比预防与老化相关的特定慢性疾病更为有效。延缓老化过程不仅可以延长寿命，而且可以延缓与老化相关疾病的发生，从而延长健康期（healthspan，即人们健康长寿的时间长短）。最近，在衰老研究中开始着重于扩大健康跨度的新领域。该领域称为「衰老科学」(geroscience)[1]。延长健康期是提升寿命的主要组成部分，定义为寿命长，但具有令人满意的健康，幸福感和生活质量[2]。现在，延长健康期的尝试着重于减缓老化背后的基本生物学过程，例如粒线体功能障碍，蛋白质稳性受损，细胞衰老，与老化相关的抗压性下降，涉及生长和细胞能量感应的机转失调，使干细胞的功能和/或生物利用度恶化，氧化压迫和炎症[3,4]。致力于延长人类寿命这一新研究领域的一部分称为「抗老化医学」，抗老化医学在过去的几年中一直是一个日益受到争议的话题[5]。衰老不一定是不可逆的，而是可以改善的，发现减缓甚至逆转老化过程的方法将是未来的挑战[5]。

有足够的证据表示抗老化干预措施将延迟和预防老化相关的疾病。一线策略是健康的生活方式，包括健康的饮食，规律运动，健康的生活方式，戒菸和戒酒。生活方式的改变可以直接影响老化的速度，并可以减轻与老化相关的疾病的负担，包括心血管疾病，癌症，骨质疏松症，关节炎，糖尿病和痴呆症等神经退化性疾病。良好的营养不仅可以增加寿命，而且可以增加生活品质。高脂饮食会导致胰岛素抗性，高血压，炎症和血管改变，所有这些都可能导致老人痴呆。高蛋白，高碳水化合物饮食会对心脏代谢健康参数产生不利影响。包括地中海饮食，DASH 饮食在内的饮食模式可改善与老化相关的健康，并减少与老化相关疾病的风险。饮食通过一组称为营养感应途径 (nutrient sensing pathways) 的细胞途径影响老化，而营养感应代谢途径中信号的改变（诱导）会影响心脏新陈代谢健康和老化[6]。缺乏运动会导致慢性疾病，包括肥胖，糖尿病，心血管疾病和老人痴呆。规律运动通过减弱老化的主要特征 ("hallmarks of aging)[7]，具有多系统抗老化作用。抽烟有许多不利的健康后果，包括糖尿病，心血管疾病，癌症，肺部疾病和老人痴呆。饮酒有害于心脏新陈代谢健康和老人痴呆。社交互动，尤其是晚年的社交互动，对于衰老

期间的大脑健康至关重要。积极和社会融合的生活方式可以预防老人痴呆症[8]。

热量限制可延缓衰老并改善心脏代谢健康，提高胰岛素敏感性，减少炎症，氧化压迫和总体发病率。动物研究表示，卡路里限制以及营养和生长信号通路的突变都可以使寿命延长30-50%。这些干预措施还可以降低与老化相关的功能丧失和疾病的患病率，包括癌症，心血管疾病和神经退化性病[9]。热量限制改善了与老化相关的心肌僵硬度，自主神经功能和骨骼肌肉的变化[10]。在人体试验研究中，证据表明，禁食疗法具有抗衰老作用。在进行隔日禁食的西班牙家庭护理居民中，与老化相关的发病率较低，寿命更长[11]。

已经发现了许多影响代谢，生长，炎症和外基因改变的重要途径，这些途径改变了老化的速度和与老化相关疾病的发生率。诸如行为，饮食和药理学方法的干预已经出现，可以调节相关的细胞内信号传导途径。这些措施包括间歇性禁食，低血糖指数饮食和蛋白质限制，抗老化药物（如 metformin, resveratrol, rapamycin, statins, beta-blockers, rennin-angiotensin-aldosterone system inhibitors 和几种抗炎药）的治疗。诸如抗高血压药，血糖调节剂和血脂调节剂之类的药物对于需要它们的人当然可以视为抗老化药物，因为它们可以抑制已知会缩短健康期和寿命的疾病。热量限制会改变人体老化的许多参数，包括影响染色体的外基因改变，激素状态（特别是胰岛素样生长因子和甲状腺激素的血清浓度），氧化压迫，炎症，粒线体功能和葡萄糖等稳性[9]。

自噬机转（"自食", autophagy）是溶酶体（lysosome，一种细胞器）的分解过程和保护机制，可消除受损的细胞器（微小的细胞成分），滞留、错误折叠的蛋白质和入侵的病原体，从而维持细胞等稳性并防止多种疾病如糖尿病，高血压，肝病，癌症，神经退化性疾病，自体免疫性疾病和感染等疾病。失能的自噬机转与老化相关的疾病有关。自噬机转可以通过保证细胞蛋白的稳定性和适当的细胞器更新来防止或减缓老化。限制热量和运动可以防止自噬机转随着年龄的增长而下降，因此可以减缓衰老进程。

免疫系统通过去除病原体和损害来维持全身健康。免疫衰老 (immune senescence) 是指先天性和

适应性免疫系统成长和功能的一系列与老化相关的恶关的恶化性变化。这导致对感染，组织损伤和癌症的无效控制。自噬机转是细胞等稳性的关键质量控制机制，并且随着年龄的增长，细胞凋亡（apoptosis，即程序性细胞死亡）和免疫衰老也随之而来。免疫衰老导致外来病原体去除效率低下和导致局部破坏，进而导致多种与老化相关的疾病。自噬机转可以延迟或恢复免疫和细胞衰老，进而可以预防或减轻与老化相关的疾病并延长健康和生命期[12]。

　　近年来，证明了居住在胃肠道中的微生细菌群在调节健康状况和寿命方面的关键作用[13,14]。该细菌群统称为肠道微生态(microbiota)或微生物组(microbiome)，意指这些细菌具有的所有基因。微生态被证明会影响宿主生物的几种重要的生理和代谢功能，从而促进终身的体内平衡。成年状的肠道微生物群建立于生命的最初3-5年，并且在余下的生命中保持相对稳定，但可能会根据生活方式，抗生素或手术干预等而改变[15,16]。健康的肠道微生态在控制新陈代谢，抵抗感染和炎症，预防自体免疫性疾病和癌症以及调节脑肠轴(brain-gut axis)相互关系中起著关键作用[17]。此外，肠道微生态会影响胃肠道疾病的风险，

例如大肠癌，炎症性肠病(inflammatory bowel disease) 和肠易激综合症 (irritable bowel syndrome)，以及一些肠外疾病，包括影响肝脏和呼吸道的疾病（支气管哮喘，过敏等）[18]。益生菌(probiotics) 可以预防和治疗这些疾病和其他疾病[17]。肠道微生态的组成会随着老化和相关疾病的结果而显著变化[19]。以微生物组为目标的干预措施不仅可以治疗与老化相关的疾病，而且可以减缓老化过程本身并促进人类健康和长寿。有大量的实验和临床证据表示，补充益生菌可以改善新陈代谢和心血管健康状况，减少炎症介质 (inflammatory mediators)，血糖水平，血压和体重指数[20]。在动物模型中，热量限制会改变肠道微生态结构，导致寿命延长。

随着年龄的增长，荷尔蒙减少（如生长激素，性激素，脱氢表雄酮（dehydroepiandrosterone，DHEA））很常见，并且与垂体，肾上腺和性腺的分泌减少有关。荷尔蒙缺乏会导致皮肤衰老，瘦体重，骨质密度，性欲和勃起功能，智力活动和情绪下降。然而，补充荷尔蒙作为「抗衰老作用」太笼统，不能作为治疗的基础。为了更好的定义老人补充荷尔蒙的确切适应症和治疗方式，有必要进行大规模临床研究

。这种替代疗法的长期安全性也应探讨。

　　老化与受损粒线体的积累有关，产生更多的活性氧自由基（reactive oxygen species，ROS），从而进一步氧化细胞内的蛋白质，脂质，DNA和RNA成分，导致氧化压迫[21,22,23]。除了引起氧化压迫损伤外，另一方面ROS亦可提供启动抗衰老反应（例如自噬机转）的激活信号，这反过来可能会限制氧化损伤的进展[24]。如果有效激活这些反应以防止ROS进一步积聚和氧化损伤，则可以维持细胞等稳性。由于抗氧化剂既有益又有害，所以单独添加抗氧化剂可能会给健康和全因死亡率带来不良后果[25]。

参考文献

1. Kennedy BK, Berger SL, Brunet A et al. Geroscience: linking aging to chronic disease. Cell 2014;159:709-13
2. Seals DR, Justice JN, La Rocca TJ. Physiological geroscience : targeting function to increase healthspan and achieve optimal longevity. J Physiol 2016;594(8):2001-24
3. Fontana L, Kennedy BK, Longo VD, Seals D, Melov S. Medical research: treating aging. Nature 2014;511:405-7
4. Kirkland JL. Translating advances from the basic biology of aging into clinical application. Exp Gerontol 2013;48:1-5
5. Anto B, Vitetta L, Cortizo F, Sali A. Can we delay aging? The biology and science of aging Ann NY Acad Sci 2005;1057:525-35
6. Zemke D et al. The mTOR pathway as a potential target for the development of therapies against neurological disease. Drug News Perspect 2007;20:495-9
7. Garatachea IV, Pareja-Galeano H, Sanchis-Gomar F et al. Exercise attenuates the major hallmarks of aging. Rejuvenation Res 2015;18(1):57-89
8. Fratiglioni L et al. An active and socially integrated lifestyle in late life might protect against dementia. Lancet Neurol 2004;3:343-53
9. Fontana L, Patridge L, Longo VP. Extending healthy life span – from yeast to humans. Science 2010;328:321-6
10. Mattison JA, Roth GS, Beasley TM et al. Impact of calorie restriction on health and survival in rhesus monkey from the IVIA Study. Nature 2012;489:318-21
11. Mercken EM, Carboneau BA, Krzysik-Walker SM, de Cabo R. Of mice and men: the benefits of calorie restriction, exercise and mimetics. Aging Res Rev 2012;11:390-8
12. Zhang H, Puleston DJ, Simon AK. Autophagy and

immune senescence. Trends Mol Med 2016;22(8):671-86
13. Biagi E, Nylund L, Candela M et al. Through aging beyond: gut microbiota and inflammatory status in seniors and centenarians. PLoS One 2010;5(5):e10667
14. Biagi E, Franceschi C, Rampelli S et al. Gut microbiota and extreme longevity. Curr Biol 2016;26(11):1480-5
15. Rodriguez JM, Murphy K, Stanton C et al. The composition of the gut microbiota throughout life, with an emphasis on early life. Microb Ecol Health Dis 2015;26:26050
16. Kashtanova DA, Popenko AS, Tkachera ON et al. Association between the gut microbiota and diet: fetal life, early childhood and further life. Nutrition 2016;32(6):620-7
17. Konturek PC, Haziri D, Brzozowski T et al. Emerging role of fecal microbiota therapy in the treatment of gastrointestinal and extra-gastrointestinal diseases. J Physiol Pharmacol 2015;66(4):483-91
18. Tojo R, Suarez A, Clemente MG et al. Intestinal microbiota in health and disease: role of bifidobacteria in gut homeostasis. World J Gastrointerol 2014;20(41):15163-76
19. Lakshminarayanan B, Stanton C, O'Toole DW, Ross RP. Compositional dynamics of the human intestinal microbiota with aging: implications for health. J Nutr Health Aging 2014;18(9):773-86
20. Thushara RM, Gangadaran S, Solati Z, Moghadassan MH. Cardiovascular benefits of probiotics: a review of experimental and clinical studies. Food Funct 2016;7(2):632-42
21. Sohal RS, Sohal BH. Hydrogen peroxide release by mitochondria increases during aging. Mech Ageing Dev 1991;57:187-202
22. Grimm S et al. Protein oxidative modifications in the aging brain: consequence for the onset of

neurodegenerative disease. Free Radic Res 2011;45:73-83
23. Nie B et al. Age-dependent accumulation of 8-oxoguanine in the DNA and RNA in various rat tissues. Oxid Med Cell Longev 2013;303181
24. Scherz-Shuval R, Elazar Z. Regulation of autophagy by ROS:physiology and pathology. Trend Biochem Sci 2011;36:30-8
25. Bjelakoric G et al. Antioxidant supplements and mortality. Curr Opin Clin Nutr Metab Care 2014;17:40-4

第四章

养生保健法：逆转疾病及老化

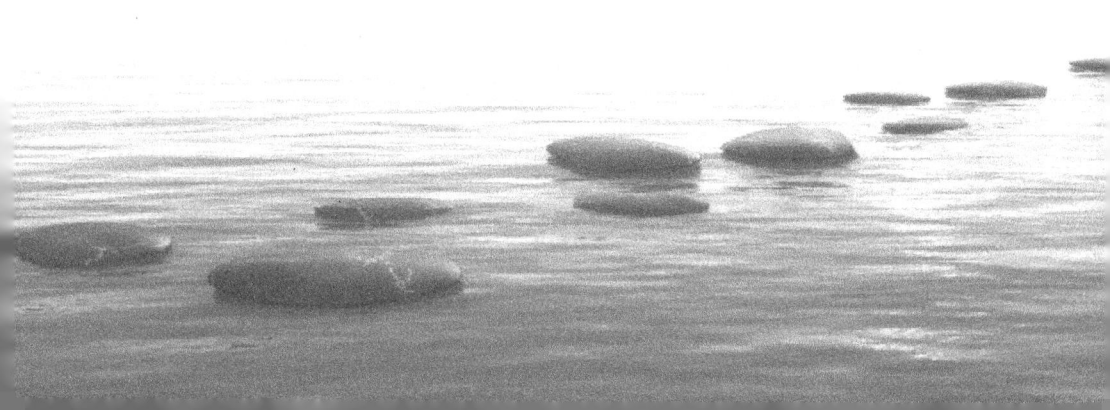

养生保健法－逆转疾病及老化

　　细胞是生命的基础单位。所有细胞含有去氧核糖核酸(deoxyribonucleic acid，DNA) 以储存遗传资讯，用以带领蛋白质合成，从而产生各种细胞独特的结构，功能及生成物。基因 (genes) 是由 DNA 组成，而基因丝毫不差地合成蛋白质 (基因表达, gene expression)。每个细胞全部的基因及 DNA 合称基因组（genome）。基因是线性排列成染色体 (chromosomes)。在多细胞生物的细胞，虽然含有相同的基因组，但其基因表达 (gene expression) 可以是不一样的。依据其环境影响，这些细胞利用其遗传资讯 (基因型, genotype) 引导其生化活动，从而产生各种细胞独特的结构，功能及生成物，从而控制生物的特征 (遗传表型, phenotype) 及功能。

　　组织 (tissue) 是细胞及细胞间物质的聚合，以执行共同工作。器官 (organ) 是不同组织以明确的比例及模式结合以执行共同工作。器官系统 (organ system) 是二至多种器官化学或/及物理的相互作用，从而提供整个生命体的生存。组织、器官及器官系统一起工作，以维持生物体内稳定环境 (亦即细胞外流体,

extracellular fluid，亦称系统性环境或因子, systemic milieu or factors)，以维持个别细胞生存需求。当体内等稳性 (homeostasis) 时，体内环境平衡最有利于细胞功能。生命体对其环境反应，它会产生调整及代偿机转，以维持身体内等稳性。生物系统是由分子、基因、细胞内小器官 (organelle)、细胞及组织、组织之间，器官之间，及器官系统之间交互作用网络建造而成。所有交互作用层次都提供生命体最终的特征 (phenotype) 及功能，以维持等稳性的系统性环境或因子。相反，系统性因子在器官系统之间，器官之间，组织之间，细胞与组织之间以及细胞之间相互作用，从而维持细胞等稳性和结构。因此，这些相互作用的网络决定了细胞的结构和功能，而细胞的结构和功能是相互作用的。换句话说，正常细胞能相互作用或引起正常的表现形态 (phenotype) 具正常因子及正常机能；反之，正常机能具正常因子或正常表现形态能相互作用或导致正常细胞结构。相反角度来看，异常细胞能相互作用或引起异常的表现形态具异常因子及异常机能；反之，异常机能具异常因子或异常表现形态，能相互作用或导致异常细胞结构。补给正常因子同时移除异常因子因此可以调整或引致正常细胞结构具正常表现形态及正常机能。此外，生物系统对环

境反应是体内等稳性的基础。越来越清楚知道上述交互作用网络内外间的联络，力图于压力情况下恢复体内等稳性，是成功抗老化方案的主要要点。同样，生理性压力如全身系统优化可以诱发代偿性适应，从而在分子，细胞，结构，组织和器官水平上维持人体的等稳性和功能，亦是成功抗老化方案的主要策略。

要维持生命，你的细胞需浸泡在提供养份及移除代谢废物的流体。如此看来，多细胞生物与单细胞生物是一致的。分别是你的身体有佰万兆细胞同时存在。不在细胞内的是细胞外液。很多是组织间液，即它占有细胞及组织间的空间。其余的是血浆，即血液中流体部分。组织间液于其浸泡的细胞及血液间交换物质。从机能上的关系看来，细胞内液及细胞外液是无间隔的，相通的。这是细胞外液或系统性环境或因子成分及容量毅然地改变会对细胞功能强烈改变的原因。

生命体无论简单或复杂并无差异。所有生命体组合成份一起作用，以维持稳定的流体环境以达所有细胞生存所需。体内每个细胞从事基础新陈代谢活动以确保其自己本身的生存。组织的细胞也从事一或多

种的活动，以提供整体的生存。个别细胞、组织、器官及器官系统共同作用以维持体内稳定环境——亦即细胞外流体或系统性环境或因子 - 以维持个别细胞的生存。

Claude Bernard 在 1878 年首次指出，活生物体的生存构造部分存在于沐浴它们的流体中（内部环境, internal environment 或细胞外液,extracellular fluid），并且所有生理重要机制（生命）都依赖于稳定的内部环境或体内平衡等稳性 (homeostasis)。[1,2]

将二只动物连体 (parabiosis) 以探讨其体内或循环因子(细胞外液) 的相互作用，最少已有 150 年的科学研究。另一种换汤不换药的技术 - 老少连体 (heterochronic parabiosis) (图一，图二) 即不同年龄的二只动物连体以探讨老化或老化相关疾病体内调整物或因子，亦有佰年科学历史。

图一： 老少连体 (heterochronic parabiosis)：年轻及年老大白鼠以手术方式连体

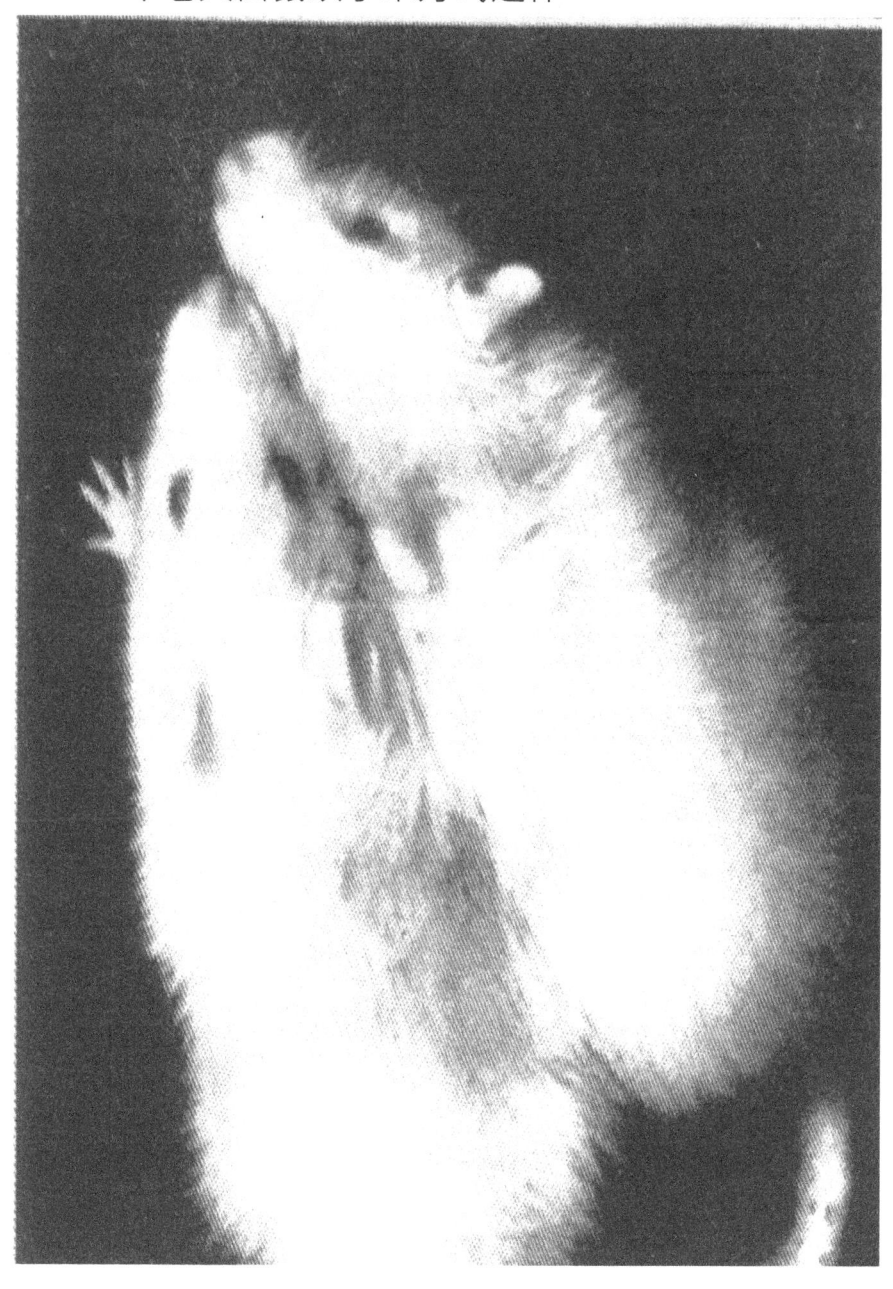

图二：老少连体 (heterochronic parabiosis)：年轻大白鼠补给年老大白鼠年轻或正常血液或因子，而同时年老大白鼠输给年轻大白鼠年老或异常血液或因子。所以年老大白鼠接受正常因子及同时移除异常因子。

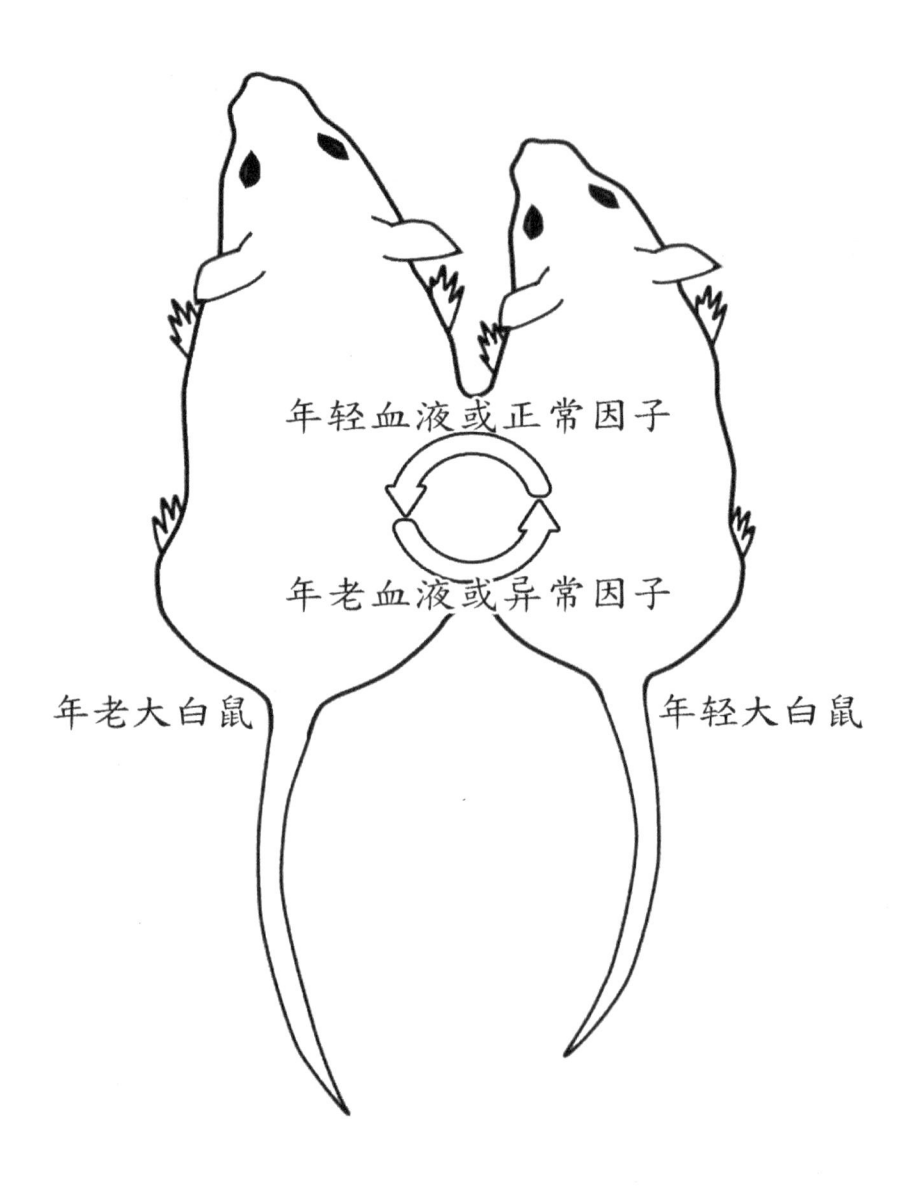

年轻血液或正常因子

年老血液或异常因子

年老大白鼠　　　　　　　　　　年轻大白鼠

连体是指以手术方式将二只活生生的动物连接在一起生活及产生单一、共有的循环系统。以此技术，二只动物连体，通常是邻接两侧腰窝，造成新的血管吻合，产生共有的血液循环。老少连体，即不同年龄的二只动物连体，能提供实验模式以探讨细胞及组织老化进行过程的体内作用，老化相关疾病的进行过程，或其他老化相关指标包括生物体寿命。已有报导，与健康动物连体，可以延长致命疾病或致命处置如辐射的实验动物生命期[3,4,5]。与健康动物连体，原发性肌肉营养不良症(muscular dystrophy)的大白鼠可以延长其生命期[6]。皮肤创伤通常愈合不良的糖尿病动物，与正常动物连体，会加速伤口愈合，加速血管生成，及修复伤口作用的发炎细胞增加。这些或其他相关的研究引发探讨老化引起的疾病，可能可以与健康、年轻连体治疗或逆转，亦可能可以延长生命期。自1950年后，已有老少连体报导老化生理及调整生命期的研究，显示年老连体动物组织作用及生命期皆有效益[7-12]。当接触年轻环境，年老的干细胞会采纳较年轻的潜能，相对，当接触年老环境，年轻的干细胞会丧失再生能力[13,14,15]。老少连体实验亦指出老年连体动物肌肉[13,14]、肝[13]、脊髓[16]、大脑[16]干细

胞功能皆被改善。与年老环境接触，年轻动物肌肉[15]及神经[16]细胞形成受抑制。

于1972年，Ludwig及Elashoff发现与同年动物比较，年老的连体动物，会因为受年轻环境反应而生命延长[10]。此老少连体模式后来应用于探讨不同组织及器官系统，老化及干细胞的生理。Conboy等应用老少连体模式，发现年轻的体内环境，可以活化年老连体动物的肝及肌肉干细胞之分子讯息路径，导致组织再生及增生[14]。Ruckn等报告年轻体内环境，可以增强大脑在经实验导致的病变恢复[17]。Salpeter等指出年老连体动物衰退的胰脏细胞增生功能（会导致糖尿病）会因为年轻环境逆转[18]。Loffredo等以老少连体动物模式指出年老连体动物的心脏肥厚及功能丧失，会因年轻体内环境而逆转[19]。Huang等报导年轻体内环境不止增强年老肾脏自噬功能(细胞清除细胞废弃物的机转以维持细胞等稳性)，更可减少年老肾脏的发炎，从而减少了肾脏组织损伤及改善肾脏老化[20]。Sidorenko等发现年轻连体动物免疫功能衰退，而年老连体动物免疫功能维持不变[21]。

体内环境是一复杂组织，免疫细胞及循环分子

或因子的储存，但其与各器官系统的联络关系仍未十分了解。有一主要问题是动物可传送的流液因子，是否在其连体动物具生理作用。年轻动物的循环因子或细胞是否能保护年老相关疾病，反之，年老动物的循环因子或细胞是否会诱发或促进年轻动物罹病。

有些哺乳动物因异常胚胎发育成单胚双胞胎，形成自然的连体动物，产生二人连体，在人类称之为连体婴。

在老少连体实验模式中，当二只动物循环系统连接在一起时，年老动物会恢复年轻[8]。怀孕可以被认为是一种特别的连体方式，其中年老动物(母亲)紧紧地连接年轻动物(胎儿)。明显地，他们的血液不是流通在一起，但不能排除他们的调整因子交换的可能。近期研究指出怀孕可能对孕妇的多种器官具有利生理作用及生命期一般延长。已经报导大白鼠怀孕会增强肝[22]及肌肉[23]再生。再者，大白鼠怀孕能保护心脏缺血损伤[24]。在心肌病病人，有一半的怀孕及分娩妇女自然恢复心脏功能[25,26]。有一种因神经发炎引起大脑损伤的多发性硬化症（multiple sclerosis）。此疾病的特征是大脑的髓鞘质(myelin)及神经间胶质

细胞 (oligodendrocyte) 发炎，引起髓鞘脱失导致大脑神经损伤及损失。PRIMS (pregnancy in multiple sclerosis)研究指出在怀孕期间，多发性硬化症病人的复发率减少[27]。再者，多产妇罹患多发性硬化症比无生育妇女少[27]。分析15,000双胞胎后显示有儿女的双胞胎(男及女)生命期比无儿女的双胞胎延长[28]。

Robo等为排除连体动物共同器官或调适作用等的影响，改利用老少血液交换系统[29]。他们指出血液交换可增强老年大白鼠肌肉修复，但对年轻大白鼠无作用；可增强老年大白鼠产生肝细胞及减少肝纤维化和脂肪肝，而年轻大白鼠肝细胞的产生则减少。再者，年老血液抑制脑细胞的产生远比年轻血液恢复脑细胞强烈。出人意料地，老少血液交换影响肌肉、肝及脑细胞的产生会于几天内发生。

血液交换用以治疗的疾病如镰状细胞贫血（sickle cell anemia）、婴儿溶血性贫血(hemolytic disease of newborn)等是常规的医疗方法[30]。血浆交换亦用于治疗血小板减少性紫斑症(thrombotic thrombocytopenic purpura)，感染性多神经炎(Guillian-Barre syndrome)等疾病[31]。这些体外的

血液交换是医界批准方法，所以能提供探讨人类老化及老化相关疾病的可行模式。

很多研究指出接触年轻血液可以改善年老组织包括骨骼肌肉，肝及大脑等功能[32,33]。再有其他研究陈述年轻血液有特别的年轻相关蛋白质活性包括 GDF11[34], TIMP2[35], oxytocin[36] 及 osteocalcin[37] 等具有部分抗老化效果。这些研究建议血液交换疗法是抑制老化及老化相关疾病精明的方法。

早期研究利用手术方法将年老及年轻大白鼠连体揭露年轻血液在年老大白鼠生命期的影响[9,11]。后来，年轻血液在年老大白鼠很多组织扮演的角色被探讨。Brack 等指出年轻血液减少年老引起的肌肉纤维化[15]。其后在老少连体或血液交换模式亦有报导肌肉骨骼干细胞能再生[29,38]。Loffredo 等利用老少连体实验指出年老大白鼠因分享年轻血液能减少心脏肥厚及心脏细胞大小[19]。因分享年轻血液，年老引起的胰脏细胞机能不全（会导致糖尿病）能够逆转[18]；并且可以改善肾脏老化[20]。经分享年轻血液，能改善年老大白鼠的骨骼恢复[39]，也能增加脑细胞生成及改善神经间传导适应性[40]。

年轻血浆扮演的角色亦被探讨。例如，年轻血浆能改善年老大白鼠神经间传导适应性，记忆及焦虑相关行为[40]。经年轻血浆治疗，年老大白鼠能改善肝细胞再生及老化[41]。经人类脐带血浆治疗，年老免疫力差的大白鼠能改善神经间传导适应性及认知表现。这指出不论任何种类，年轻血浆具恢复年轻机能[35]。再者，人类脐带血浆亦能改善年老大白鼠老年痴呆及认知表现[42]。

年轻血液里的因子扮演的角色被探讨。年轻大白鼠接受年老血液CCL11或B2M因子后产生记忆力衰退及脑细胞生成减少[16,43]。相对地，年老大白鼠接受年轻血液因子如GDF11会改善心脏肥厚，肌肉再生，脑血管及脑细胞生成[19,33,37]。年轻血液里oxytocin因子增加，它可以改善年老引起的肌肉再生衰退[35]。注入生长释出激素(growth hormone releasing hormone)，可改善动物及人类年老引起的认知衰退[44,45]。TIMP2因子在年轻大白鼠血液及人类脐带血浆上升，它能增加年老大白鼠神经间传导适应性及改善学习及记忆机能[35]。Osteocalcin因子能改善年老大白鼠记忆及焦虑行为[37]。这些结果指出多方面的年轻（正常）及年老（异常）因子在不同的器官

间相对地传达年轻及年老血液的作用。这些血液循环的因子深切地影响组织及器官疾病和老化，及逆转老化的结构及分子机转。但是，很难识别所有正常和异常因子。

所以，近期研究认定老化及老化相关疾病可以逆转的实例；老化及组织病理是可以即时的，快速的，有效的从年老逆转至年轻状态。

早期这些连体动物及血浆交换实验鼓励简单的将年轻人血浆输至年老及年老相关疾病病患探讨。PLASMA (the plasma for Alzheimer's symptom amelioration) 研究评估利用年轻成人 (18 至 30 岁) 血浆治疗老年痴呆老年病人的可行性及安全性。但发现只有极少有利治疗效果 [46]。

生命的单位是细胞，具有结构 (structure) 及机能 (function)。结构及机能是互相关联的。正常细胞能调整或引起正常的表现形态 (phenotype) 具正常因子及正常机能；反之，正常机能具正常因子或正常表现形态能调整或导致正常细胞结构。相反角度来看，异常细胞能调整或引起异常的表现形态具异常因子及

异常机能；反之，异常机能具异常因子或异常表现形态，能调整或导致异常细胞结构。补给正常因子同时移除异常因子因此可以调整或引致正常细胞结构具正常表现形态及正常机能。这与老少连体实验模式相似。年老连体动物接受年轻连体动物的年轻或正常因子，同时亦输出其年老或异常因子到年轻连体动物，所以相对地移除其年老或异常因子。这模式是经实验证实，能逆转疾病及老化。因此最佳的养生保健法是补给正常因子如健康饮食，运动，全身优化等。同时亦移除异常因子如停止吸菸，饮酒，消除污染物，解决心脏及代谢因素等的有利循环 (advantageous cycle)(图三)。这有利循环可以调整异常，不健康或年老细胞而导回正常，健康或年轻细胞，从而逆转疾病及老化，改善健康期及生命期。

图三： 补给正常因子 (如全身优化、健康饮食、规律运动等) 及同时移除异常因子 (如不吸烟、不喝酒、不吸毒、避免压力等) 的有利循环。此养生保健法可逆转疾病及老化。

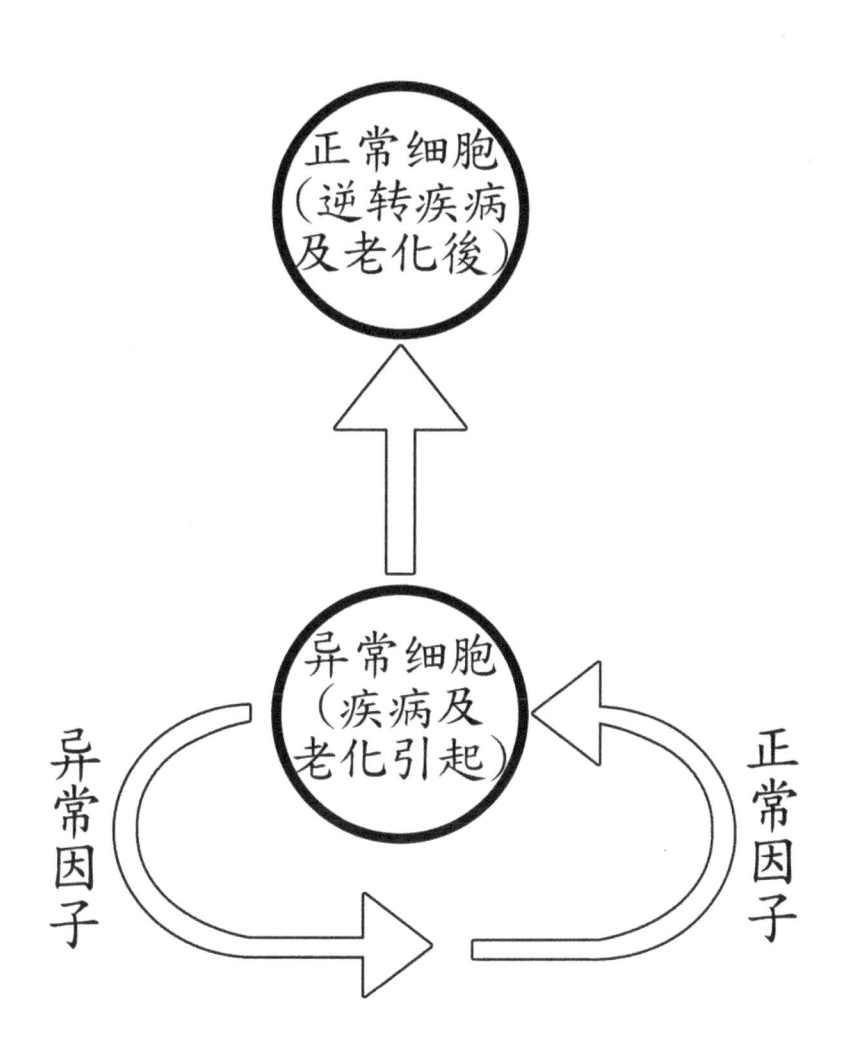

到目前为止，几乎不可能将老少连体模式，频繁的血液或血浆交换输血，补给所有正常因子及移除所有异常因子的方法作为人类的抗衰老策略或养生保健法。

众所周知，压力会导致释放因子于系统循环中以及局部中枢和周边组织内[47]。最近，证明了之前所述心脏优化能产生心脏保护性或正常因子。实验已经指出，來自经过心脏优化的动物的血浆可转移到其他动物以及在其他物种之间，用于保护心脏，表示血液循环中有心脏保护性（或正常）因子[48-51]。心脏优化和老少连体的共同联系或机制是「细胞外液」。心脏优化是一种压力，会释出因子到细胞外液。将年老和年轻动物连体(老少连体)是细胞外液中因子的交换。两者都影响细胞外液。心脏优化是对心脏有压力。心脏细胞在压力下引起代偿性适应，维持身体的等稳性和内部环境，即细胞外液，也称为系统性环境或因子。利用轻微短暂及生理性的心肌缺氧，心脏优化产生适应或代偿机转，包括激活神经内分泌系统[52,53]，心脏重塑[54]及其他事件如: 氧化作用[54]，内皮细胞分泌的血管收缩素，一氧化氮，发炎诱发因子，生长因子等。这些机转补给正常因子如: 激活交感神经及肾素-

血管收缩素-醛固酮系统 (rennin-angiotensin-aldosterone system)[52,53]，激活心脏修复及心脏重塑所需的发炎因子[54]，影响心脏细胞生态[52]，保护蛋白质产生[55]，激活细胞内酶[56]，抑制粒线体死亡[56]，一氧化氮等[56]。同时这些机转亦移除异常因子如自由基[52]，心脏缺血再灌流损伤[57]，减少心肌梗塞范围[58]，心脏凋亡机转（apoptosis，即程序性细胞死亡）[58]，提升自噬机能 (autophagy，细胞清除细胞废弃物的机转以维持细胞等稳性) 等[53]。此外，表一总结了心脏优化和老少连体模式对心脏功能的有益影响。其研究指标和结果相对相似。因此，心脏优化和老少连体模式是相关的。

表一：心脏优化及老少连体模式对心脏功能的益处

第 2.2 章

研究论文	实验模式	指标	结果
Murray et al,1986[10]	心脏前准备作用；狗	组织	减少心梗范围
Sumeray & Yellon,1998[14]	心脏前准备作用；大白鼠离体心脏	组织	减少心梗范围
Schott et al,1990[15]	心脏前准备作用；猪	组织	减少心梗范围
Cave & Hearse,1991[16]	心脏前准备作用；大白鼠离体心脏	主动脉血流	改善心脏功能
Shiki & Hearse,1987[17]	心脏前准备作用；大白鼠离体心脏	心律不整	减少缺血性心律不整
Vegh et al,1992[18]	心脏前准备作用；大白鼠及狗	心律不整	减少缺血性心律不整

研究			
Kloner et al,1995[22]	心脏前准备作用；心肌梗塞病人	心肌酶值；临床事件	减少心梗范围，住院并发症及死亡
Leslay & Beach,2003[23]	心脏前准备作用；心导管病人	临床事件	减少住院并发症及死亡
Walsch et al,2008[24]	心脏前准备作用；心脏手术病人	临床事件	减少心律不整，强心剂量及加护病房时间
Hansen et al,2010[25]	心脏前准备作用；心导管病人	心肌酶值；心脏射血分数	减少心梗范围；提升心脏射血分数
Khan et al,2014[26]	心脏后准备作用；心导管病人	心肌酶值；影像；心脏射血分数	减少心肌损伤；改善心脏功能
Staat et al,2005[27]	心脏后准备作用；心导管病人	心肌酶值；影像	减少心梗范围

Yang et al,2007 [28]	心脏后准备作用：心导管病人	心肌酶值；影像	减少心梗范围及长期保护
Thielmann et al,2013 [30]	心脏间接准备作用：心脏手术病人	心肌酶值；1.54 年死亡率	减少心梗范围及改善预后
Hode et al,2009 [31]	心脏间接准备作用：心导管病人	心肌酶值；临床事件	减少心梗范围，住院并发症及改善预后
Davis et al,2013 [32]	心脏间接准备作用：心导管病人	心肌酶值；临床事件	减少心梗范围，短及长期并发症
Crimi et al,2013 [33]	心脏间接准备作用：心导管病人	心肌酶值；影像	减少心梗范围

第 4 章

Loffredo et al,2013 [19]	老少连体；大白鼠	组织	心脏肥大及心脏细胞大小复原

Xiao et al,2013[24]	怀孕作为老少连体模式；大白鼠	聚合酶链反应(PCR)；western blot；免疫荧光染色	防止心脏缺血性损伤；激活心脏母细胞
Felker et al,2000[25]	怀孕作为老少连体模式；心肌病变病人	回顾性统计分析	恢复心脏功能
Katsimpardi et al,2014[34]	老少连体；血清GDF 11因子；大白鼠	组织；影像	诱发血管重塑；逆转心脏肥大

利用轻微短暂的之前运动，肺优化产生「暖身」(warm-up) 或「闪过、避开」(running through) 现象，可以减轻之后持续运动产生的气管收缩反应。这不反应期补给正常因子如气管重塑 (airway remodeling)，改善心肺功能，释出保护因子如 prostaglandin 等。同时这「暖身」现象移除异常因子如自由基，发炎，气管水肿，减少发炎细胞诱发因子 (mast cell mediators)，减少释出神经胜肽 (neuropeptides)，减少气管肌肉反应等 [59]。

利用节食 (calorie restriction) 及间歇性断食 (intermittent fasting)，肠优化产生代偿机转包括提升细胞的适应或防御机转，肠重塑及减少氧化作用，粒线体机能障碍及发炎，调整肠凋亡及自噬机能 [60-63]。这些机转补给正常因子如改善疾病指标 [64]，改善胰岛素敏感度 [65]，影响内分泌系统 [66]，改善粒线体功能，肠道重塑，调整肠凋亡及自噬机能等 [60-63]。这些机转亦同时移除异常因子如减少血糖及脂肪 [67]，减少氧化及发炎作用 [68]，减少心脏损伤及梗塞 [69]，减少血管硬化等 [70]。

所以全身系统优化能产生适应，防卫及代偿机

转，能同时补给正常因子及移除异常因子，导致优化，保护健康及很多器官和组织如神经系统，心脏，肺，肠胃，肾，肌肉等机能。

规律运动有多重器官系统抗老化作用。运动可以启动心脏优化，也可能产生心脏保护(或正常)因子[71]。规律运动补给正常因子如一氧化氮[72,73]，血管生成(angiogenesis)、自噬功能、粒线体生成(mitochondrial biogenesis)、神经细胞产生[74]、神经因子(neurotrophic factors)[75,76,77]、调整染色体终端长度(telomere length)[78]、遗传调整[79]、活化营养感应路径[80]、胰岛素感应性[81]、干细胞增生及移动[82]、调控免疫功能等[83]。规律运动移除异常因子如血管内皮异常[72,73]，自由基[72,73]，脂肪[83]，自主神经失调[84]，粒线体不稳定[85]，衰老细胞[86]，发炎[86]，心脏代谢因素等。

饮食是影响健康，疾病及寿命的重要生活方式。饮食直接影响养份摄取及循环系统中生长因子及荷尔蒙值，从而影响全身组织等稳性[87]。干细胞的基本作用是在生命期对生长及再生需求产生功能，这些过程都是基本上与营养改变相关[88]。饮食可以改变在体内

环境中如糖，胺基酸及脂肪酸的成份，而影响很多主要体内生化机转。营养感应路径 (nutrient-sensing signaling pathways) 受营养改变反应而指挥细胞及生命体的新陈代谢，对调控健康及生命期有莫大关系。间歇性断食(intermittent fasting) 可以启动心脏优化，也可能产生心脏保护 (或正常) 因子 [89,90,91]。健康饮食补给正常因子如养分，植物化学物(phytochemicals)，能量，自噬功能(autophagy)，神经传导介质 (neurotransmitters)，神经细胞产生[92,93,94]，一氧化氮(nitric oxide)，遗传调控(epigenetic modulations)[95] 等。健康饮食移除异常因子如自由基，胰岛素抗性，发炎，血管硬化，血管内皮异常 [96,97]，心脏代谢因素，血管僵硬等 [98]。

如果您有老人病或综合性的疾病，现代医学可以应用移除异常因子及补给正常因子来治疗甚至逆转疾病。譬如，如果您有细菌性肺炎，抗生素可以扼杀或移除侵入的细菌及肺炎病变 (移除异常因子)，而肺能恢复等稳性及机能 (补给正常因子)。如果您患有冠心病，就以心绞痛药物，心导管或心血管手术以调整或移除心血管的阻塞而让心脏恢复正常等稳性及机能。同样地，抗血压药降低血压 (移除异常因子) 及维持

正常血压 (补给正常因子)。抗血脂药降低血液中三甘油脂及胆固醇而维持正常血脂值。糖尿病药物降低血糖及减轻糖尿病并发症。静脉注射硝酸甘油 (nitroglycerin) 提升一氧化氮,可以启动心脏优化,也可能产生心脏保护 (或正常) 因子 [99]。

现代医学(包括中医)能治疗或逆转一佰年前可能令我们死亡的很多疾病或创伤。无疑问地,如降血压药,降血糖药及降血脂药等对需要的病人而言都可称为抗老化治疗。因为这些药物抑制会减少健康及生命期的疾病。

利用现代医学、饮食、运动、生活方式改变及全身系统优化,以提供正常因子及同时移除异常因子,这种养生保健法可以逆转疾病及老化,与老少连体模式类似。特别地,由于全身系统优化会导致细胞处于轻度生理性的压迫,细胞会通过恢复等稳性维持体内稳定环境或系统性环境,及增强其适应力以应对压迫,可能会抵抗或逆转疾病及老化。由于功能和结构是相互联系的,因此异常或年老细胞也可以逆转为正常或年轻细胞（图三）。实际上,我们可以利用现代医学,健康饮食,规律运动,健康的生活方式和

全身系统优化来实行养生保健，从而享受健康美好的生活。

很明显，养生保健法是个人化的，视个人疾病，健康及经济条件，以及个人偏好而定。此外，如果我们治疗老年相关疾病，我们同时亦治疗老化。反过来说，如果我们治疗老化，我们同时亦治疗老年相关疾病及综合性的疾病。养生保健法的目的是治疗甚而逆转老化，老年相关疾病及综合性疾病。如果我们不生病及不老化，便是健康。老少连体实验摸式证实，养生保健，就是逆转疾病及老化。

简而言之，养生保健医学 (healthy medicine) 是使您保持健康的医学。健康是指您没有疾病，也没有老化。养生保健法是指逆转疾病及老化。养生保健医学涉及许多学科，例如老化，抗老化，老年科学，老年医学，预防医学，基础和临床科学等。从实际意义上讲，养生保健医学强调针对疾病和老化逆转的养生保健法 (healthy regimens)，如老少连体模式（老年和幼年动物连体以研究老化和抗老化机转）证实。总而言之，养生保健医学是诊断、预防、治疗及逆转疾病及老化的科学或医疗业务。

参考文献

1. Bernard C. Les Phenomenes de la Vic. Paris 1878, two vols.
2. Cannon WR. Organization for physiological homeostasis. Physiol Rev 1929;9(3):399-431
3. Finerty JC, Binhammer R, Schnerder M. Protection of irradiated rats by parabiosis. Tex Rep Biol Med 1952;10:496-500
4. Warrens S, Chute RN, Farrington EM. Protection of the hematopoietic system by parabiosis. Lab Invest 1960;9:191-8
5. Carroll IM, Kimeldorf DJ. Mechanisms of protection against gastrointestinal and hematopoietic radiation lethality by parabiosis. Radiat Res 1969;39:770-6
6. Hall CE, Hall O, Neris AH. Prolongation of survival by parabiosis in strain 129 dystrophic mice. Am J Physiol 1959;196:110-2
7. Pietramaggiori G, Scherer SS, Alperovich M et al. Improved cutaneous healing in diabetic mice exposed to healthy peripheral circulation. J Invest Dermatol 2009;129:2265-74
8. Pope F, Lunsford W, McCay CM. Experimental prolongation of the life span. J Chronic Dis 1956;4:153-8
9. McCay CM, Pope F, Lunsford W, Sperlig G, Sambharaphol P. Parabiosis between old and young rats. Gerontologia 1957;1:7-17
10. Lunsford WR, McCay CM, Lupien PJ, Pope FE, SperlingG. Parabiosis as a method for studying factors which affect aging in rats. Gerontologia 1963;7:1-8
11. Ludwig FC, Elashoff RM. Mortality in syneneic rat parabionts of different chronological age. Trans NY Acad Sci 1972;34:582-7
12. Sidorenko AV, Gubrii IB, Andrianova LF, Macsijuk TV, Butenko GM. Functional rearrangement of lymphohemopoietic system in heterochronically

parabiosed mice. Mech Ageing Dev 1986;36:41-56
13. Butenko GM. Active mechanisms of dysfunction in the process of aging. Vestn Adad Med Nauk SSSR 1990;2:0-23
14. Conboy IM, Conboy MJ, Wagers AJ et al. Rejuvenation of aged progenitor cells by exposure to a young systemic environment. Nature 2005;433:760-4
15. Brack AS, Conboy MJ, Roy S et al. Increased Wnt signaling during aging alters muscle stem cell fate and increases fibrosis. Science 2007;317:807-10
16. Villeda SA, Luo J, Mosher KI et al. The aging systemic milieu negatively regulated neurogenesis and cognitive function. Nature 2011;477:90-4
17. Ruckh JM et al. Rejuvenation of regeneration in the aging central nervous system. Cell Stem cell 2012;10:96-103
18. Salpeter SJ, Khalaileh A, Weinberg-Corem N et al. Systemic regulation of the age-related decline of pancreatic B-cell replication. Diabetes 2013;62(8):2843-8
19. Loffredo FS, Steinhauser ML, Jay SM et al. Growth differentiation factor 11 is a circulating factor that reverses age-related cardiac hypertrophy. Cell 2013;153:.828-39
20. Huang Q, Ning Y, Liu D et al. A young blood environment decreases aging of senile mice kidneys. J Gerontol A Biol Sci Med Sci 2018;73(4):421-8
21. Sidorenko AV, Gubrii IB, Andrianova LF, Macsijuk TV, Butenko GM. Functional rearrangement of lymphohemopoietic system in heterochronically parabiosed mice. Mechan Ageing Development 1986;36:41-56
22. Gielchinsky Y, Laufer N, Weitman E et al. Pregnancy restores the regenerative capacity of the aged liver via activation of an mTORCI-controlled hyperplasia/hypertrophy switch. Genes Dev 2010;24:543-8
23. Falick Michaeli T, Laufer N, Sagir JY et al. The rejuvenating effect of pregnancy on muscle regeneration.

Aging Cell 2015;14:698-700
24. Xiao J, Li J, Xu T et al. Pregnancy-induced physiological hypertrophy protects against cardiac ischemia-reperfusion injury. Int J Clin Exp Pathol 2013;7:229-35
25. Felker GM, Thompson RE, Hare JM et al. Underlying causes and long-term survival in patients with initially unexplained cardiomyopathy. N Eng J Med 2000;342:1077-1084
26. Ro A, Frishman WH. Peripartum cardiomyopathy. Cardiol Rev 2006;14:35-42
27. Vukusic S, Hutchinson M, Hours M et al. Pregnancy and multiple sclerosis (the PRIMS study): Clinical predictors of post-partum relapse. Brain 2004;127:1353-60
28. Chereji E, Gatz M, Pedersen NL, Prescott CA. Reexaming the association between fertility and longevity: testing the disposable soma theory in a modern human sample of twins. J Gerontol A Biol Sci Med Sci 2013;68:499-509
29. Rebo J, Mehdipour M, Gathwala R et al. A single heterochronic blood exchange reveals rapid inhibition of multiple tissues by old blood. Nat Comm 2016;7:13363
30. Smits-Wintjens VE et al. Neonatal morbidity after exchange transfusion for red cell alloimmune hemolytic disease. Neonatology 2013;103:141-7
31. Von Baeyer H. Plasmapheresis in immune hematology: review of clinical outcome data with respect to evidence-based medicine and clinical experience. Ther Apher Dial 2003;7:127-40
32. Castellano JM, Kirby ED, Wyss-Coray T. Blood-borne revitalization of the aged brain. JAMA Neurol 2015;72:1191-4
33. Wyss-Coray T. Aging, neurodegeneration and brain rejuvenation. Nature 2016;539:180-6
34. Katsimpardi L, Litterman NK, Schein PA et al. Vascular and neurogenic rejuvenation of the aging mouse brain by young systemic factors. Science 2014;344:630-4

35. Castellano JM, Mosher KI, Abbey RJ et al. Human umbilical cord plasma proteins revitalize hippocampal function in aged mice. Nature 2017;544:488-92
36. Elab C, Cousin W, Upadhyayula P et al. Oxytocin is an aged-specific circulating hormone that is necessary for muscle maintenance and regeneration. Nat Commun 2014;5:4082
37. Khriman L, Obri A, Ramos-Brossier M et al. Gpr158 mediates osteocalcin's regulation of cognition. J Exp Med 2017;214:2859-73
38. Sinha M, Jang YC, Oh J et al. Restoring systemic GDF11 levels reverses age-related dysfunction in mouse skeletal muscle. Science 2014;344:649-52
39. Baht GS, Silkstone D, Vi L et al. Exposure to a youthful circulation rejuvenates bone repair through modulation of beta-catenin. Nat Commun 2015;6:7131
40. Villeda SA, Plambeck KE, Middeldorp J et al. Young blood reverses age-related impairments in cognitive function and synaptic plasticity in mice. Nat Med 2014;20:659-63
41. Liu A, Guo E, Yang J et al. Young plasma reverses age-dependent alterations in hepatic function through the restoration of autophagy. Aging Cell 2018;17
42. Habid A, Hou H, Mori T et al. Human umbilical cord blood serum-derived alpha-secretase: functional testing in Alzheimer's disease mouse models. Cell Transplant 2018;27:438-55
43. Smith LK, He Y, Park JS et al. Beta-2 microglobulin is a systemic pro-aging factor that impairs cognitive function and neurogenesis. Nat Med 2015;21:932-7
44. Baker LD, Barsness SM, Borson S et al. Effects of growth hormone releasing hormone on cognitive function in adults with mild cognitive impairment and healthy older adults: results of a controlled trial. Arch Neurol 2012;69:1420-9

45. Thornton PL, Ingram RL, Sontag WE. Chronic (D-Ala2)-growth hormone releasing hormone administration attenuates age-related deficits in spatial memory. J Gerontol A Biol Sci Med Sci 2000;55:B106-12
46. Kaiser J. Blood from young people does little to reverse Alzheimer's in first test. Science 2017;DOI:10.1126/Science.aar3723
47. Shimizu,M., Tropak,M., Diaz,R.J. et al.,2009. Transient limb ischemia remotely preconditions through a humoral mechanism acting directly on the myocardium: evidence suggesting cross-species protection. Clin. Sci. (Lond.) 117(5),191-200.
48. Shimizu,M., Tropak,M., Diaz,R.J. et al.,2009. Transient limb ischemia remotely preconditions through a humoral mechanism acting directly on the myocardium: evidence suggesting cross-species protection. Clin. Sci. (Lond.) 117(5),191-200.
49. Leung,C.H.,Wang,L., Nielsen,J.M.et al., 2014. Remote cardioprotection by transfer of coronary effluent from ischemic preconditioned rabbit heart preserves mitochondrial integrity and function via adenosine receptor activation. Cardiovas. Drugs Ther. 28(1),7-17.
50. Surendra,H., Diaz,R.J.,Harvey,K. et al.,2013. Interaction of delta and kappa opioid receptors with adenosine A1 receptors mediates cardioprotection by remote ischemic preconditioning. J. Mol. Cell. Cardiol. 60,142-50
51. Skyschally,A., Gent,S., Amanakis,G., et al.,2015. Across-species transfer of protection by remote ischemic preconditioning with species-specific myocardial signal transduction by reperfusion injury salvage kinase and survival activating factor enhancement pathways. Cir. Res. 117(3),279-88
52. Mann DL. Basic mechanisms of disease progression in the failing heart: the role of excessive adrenergic drive. Prog Cardiovas Ds 1998;41(suppl 1):1-8

53. Dell'Italia L, Sabis A. Activation of the rennin-angiotensin system in hypertrophy and heart failure. In Mann DL (ed): Heart failure: A companion to Baunwald's Heart Disease. Philadephia, Saunders 2004;pp 129-143
54. Grieve DJ, Shah AM. Oxidative stress in heart failure. More than just damage. Eur Heart J 2003;24:2161
55. Shen YT, Depre C, Yan L et al. Repetitive ischemia by coronary stenosis induces a novel window of ischemic preconditioning. Cir 2008;118:1961-9
56. Heusch G. Cardioprotection: chances and challenges of its translation to the clinic. Lancet 2013;381:166-75
57. Murry CE, Jennings RB, Reimer KA. Preconditioning with ischemia: a delay of lethal cell injury in ischemic myocardium. Cir 1986;74:1124
58. Piot CA, Padmanaban D, Ursell PC et al. Ischemic preconditioning decreases apoptosis in rat hearts in vivo. Cir 1997;96:1598
59. Larsson J, Anderson SD, Dahlen SE, Dahlen B. Refractoriness to exercise challenges: a review of the mechanisms old and new. Immunol Allergy Clin N Am 2013;33:329-45
60. Aly KB, Piplciu JL, Hinson WG et al. Chronic calorie restriction induces stress proteins in the hypothalamus of rats. Mech Ageing Dev 1994;76:11-23.
61. Ehrenfried JA, Evers BM, Chu KV, Townsend CM, Thompson JC. Calorie restriction increases the expression of heat shock protein in the gut. Ann Surg 1996;223:592-7.
62. Doy Y, Grepersen S, Ahao J et al. Morphometric and biomechanical intestinal remodeling induced by fasting in rats. Digestive Ds Sci 2002;47(5):1158-68.
63. Marzetti E, Wholgemuth SE, Anton SD et al. Cellular mechanisms of cardioprotection by calorie restriction: state of the science and future perspectives. Clin Geriatr Med 2009;25:715-32.

64. Most J, Tosti V, Redman LM, Fontana L. Calorie restriction in humans: an update. Aging Res Rev 2017;39:36-45
65. Lu J et al. Alternate day fasting impacts the brain insulin-signaling pathway of young adult male C57BL/6 mice. J Neurochem 2011;117(1):154-63
66. Wan R, Camaridola S, Mattson MP. Intermittent fasting deprivation improves cardiovascular and neuroendocrine responses to stress in rats. J Nutri 2003;133:1921-9
67. Walford RL, Weber L, Pauor S. Calorie restriction and aging as viewed from biosphere2. Receptor 1995;5(1):29-33
68. Faris MAE, Jahrami HA, Obaideen NA, Madkour MI. Impact of diurnal intermittent fasting during Ramadan on inflammatory and oxidative stress markers in healthy people: systemic review and metaanalysis. J Nutr Intermediary Meta 2019;15:18-26.
69. Ahmet I, Wan R, Mattson MP, Lakatta EG, Talan M. Cardioprotection by intermittent fasting in rats. Cir 2005;112:3115-21
70. Fontana L, Meyer TE, Klein S, Holloszy JO. Long-term calorie restriction is highly effective in reducing the risk for atherosclerosis in humans. Proc Natl Acad Sci USA 2004;101:6659-63.
71. Lambiase, P.D., Edwards, R.J., Cusack, M.R. et al., 2003. Exercise-induced ischemia initiates the second window of protection in humans independent of collateral recruitment. J.A.C.C. 41,1174-82.
72. DeSouza CA, Shapiro LF, Clevenger CM et al. Regular aerobic exercise prevents and restores age-related declines in endothelium-dependent vasodilation in healthy men. Cir 2000;102:1351-7
73. Gielen S, Sandri M, Erbs S, Adams V. Exercise-induced modulation of endothelial nitric oxide production. Curr Pharmacent Biotech 2011;12:1375-84
74. Craig TJ, Dispenza MC. Benefits of exercise in asthma. Ann Allergy Asthma Immunol 1994;26:951-6

75. Radak Z, Hart N, Sarga L et al. Exercise plays a preventive role against Alzheimer's disease. J Alzheimers Dis 2010;20:777-83
76. Kuaepen K, Goekint M, Heyman EM, Meensen R. Neuroplasticity- exercise-induced response of peripheral brain-derived neurotrophic factor: A systematic review of experimental studies in human subjects. Sports Med 2010;40:765-801
77. Neeper SA, Gomez-Pinilla F, Choi J, Cotman CW. Physical activity increases mRNA for brain-derived neurotrophic factor and nerve growth factor in rat brain. Brain Res 1996;726:49-56
78. Cherkas LF, Hunkin JL, Kato BS et al. The association between physical activity in leisure time and leukocyte telomere length. Arch Intern Med 2008;168:154-8
79. Ntanasis-Stathopoulos J, Tzanninis JG, Philippon A, Koutsilieris M. Epigenetic regulation on gene expression induced by physical exercise. J Musculoskelet Neuronal Interact 2013;13:133-46
80. Coiro V, Volpi R, Gramellini D et al. Effect of physical t4raining on age-related reduction of GH secretion during exercise in normally cycling women. Maturitas 2010;65:392-5
81. Fujita S, Rasmussen BB, Cadenas JG et al. Aerobic exercise overcomes the age-related insulin resistance of muscle protein metabolism by improving endothelial function and Akt/mammalian target of rapamycin signaling. Diabetes 2007;56:1615-22
82. Fiuza-Luces C, Delmiro A, Soares-Miranda L et a. Exercise training can induce cardiac autophagy and at end-stage chronic conditions: Insights from a graft-versus-host-disease mouse model. Brain Behav Immun 2014;39:56-60
83. Lancaster GI, Febbraio MA. The immunomodulating role of exercise in metabolic disease. Trend Immuno 2014;35(6):262-9

84. Seals DR, Dinenno FA. Collateral damage: Cardiovascular consequences of chronic sympathetic activation in human aging. Am J Physiol Heart Cir Physiol 2004;287:H1895-1905
85. Safdar A, Bourgeois JM, Ogborn DI et al. Endurance exercise rescues progeroid aging and induces systemic mitochondrial rejuvenation in mDNA mutator mice. Proc Natl Acad Sci USA 2011;108:4135-40
86. Bigley AB, Spielmann G, LaVoy EC, Simpson RJ. Can exercise-related improvements in immunity influence cancer prevention and prognosis in the elderly? Maturitas 2013;76:51-6
87. Rafalski VA, Manchini E, Brunet A. Energy metabolism and energy-sensing pathways in mammalian embryonic and adult stem cell fate. J Cell Sci 2012;125:5597-5608
88. Signer RA, Morrison SJ. Mechanisms that regulate stem cell aging and life span. Cell Stem Cell 2013;12:152-165
89. Ahmet I, Wan R, Mattson MP, Lakatta EG, Talan M. Cardioprotection by intermittent fasting in rats. Cir 2005;112:3115-21.
90. Godar RJ, Ma X, Liu H et al. Repetitive stimulation of autophagy-lysosome machinery by intermittent fasting preconditions the myocardium to ischemia-reperfusion injury. Autophagy 2015;11:1537-60.
91. Katare RG, Kakinuma Y, Arikwa M, Yamasaki F, Sato T. Chronic intermittent fasting improves the survival following large myocardial ischemia by activation of BDNF/VEGF/D13K signaling pathway. J Mol Cell Cardiol 2009;46:405-12.
92. Kiliaan AJ, Arnoldussen IA, Gustafson DR. Adipokines: a link between obesity and dementia? Lancet Neurol 2014;13:913-23

93. Jansen D, Zerbi V, Janssen CI et al. Impact of a multi-nutrient diet on cognition, brain metabolism, hemodynamics and plasticity in apoE4 carrier and apoE knockout mice. Brain Struct Funct 2014;219:1841-68
94. Zerbi V, Jansen D, Wiesmann M et al. Multinutrient diets improve cerebral perfusion and neuroprotection in a murine model of Alzheimer's disease. Neurobiol Aging 2014;35:600-13
95. Garcia-Segura L, Perez-Andrade M, Miranda-Rios J. The emerging role of microRNAs in the regulation of gene expression by nutrients. J Nutrigenet Nutrigenomics 2013;6(1):16-31
96. Basu A, Devaraj S, Jialal I. Dietary factors that promote or retard inflammation. Arterioscler Thromb Vasc Biol 2006;26:995-1001
97. Bullo M, Casas-Agusteuch P, Amigo-Correig P, Aranceta J, Salas-Salvado J. Inflammation, obesity and comorbidities: the role of diet. Public Health Nutr 2007;10(10A):1164-72
98. LaRocca TJ, Martens CR, Seals DR. Nutrition and other lifestyle influences on arterial aging. Ageing Res Review 2017;39:106-119
99. Leesar, M.A., Stoddard, M.F., Dawn, B. et al., 2001. Delayed preconditioning-mimetic action of nitroglycerin in patients undergoing coronary angioplasty. Cir 103,2935-41.

CPSIA information can be obtained
at www.ICGtesting.com
Printed in the USA
BVHW051720050223
657834BV00004B/264

9 786267 105344